G000162913

"Bariatric Surgery Made Easy:

Your Guide For A Successful Journey"

Maher El Chaar, MD
Copyright © 2020 Maher El Chaar, MD
All rights reserved.
ISBN: 9798649439275

DEDICATION

I would like to dedicate this book to my family, above all my lovely and inspirational wife Judy, my daughters Celine and Ella, and my son Fares. Thank you for your unconditional love and support.

CONTENTS

ACKNOWLEDGMENTS

I would like to acknowledge my patients who have trusted me with their lives—you have truly honored and humbled me by choosing me to accompany you on your journey. This book is dedicated to you!

I also forward a heartfelt acknowledgment to all my amazing staff. They work passionately and tirelessly every day to help our patients do their best and achieve their goals!

INTRODUCTION

Obesity is not only becoming a major problem in the United States but in other countries too. There are many reasons why obesity is becoming a pandemic, but we won't be discussing them in this book. In the past ten years, I have taken care of thousands of patients who suffer from obesity and other associated diseases and I have learned firsthand what is important for my patients to know before and after surgery. I wrote my first book few years ago to help my patients understand what bariatric surgery is and what to expect before and after surgery. Given the recent advancements in bariatric surgery, especially with the introduction of robotic surgery, I elected to write a second book to keep my patients updated and well informed.

This is not meant to be a detailed textbook of surgery or a review of the literature but rather an accessible handbook for patients to refer to when they have a specific question. The book was written in a simple format and is divided into different chapters, each of which answers a simple question using a straightforward style without the use of complicated or confusing medical or technical terms. The book includes fifty Q&As that cover the most important questions about bariatric surgery. This new book includes newly released information on robotic surgery, obesity in children and adolescents, weight loss medications, and few other important topics that were not included in the first book. If you have a question and you are looking for a quick and easy answer you can just go to the specific chapter instead of reading the entire book. Many of my patients ask the same questions in different ways, so I have developed the habit of answering the same questions in different styles. This means you will notice that some information is repeated in different chapters—this is just to drive the message home.

If you are reading this book then you either had surgery or are considering bariatric surgery in the near future. Either way, I want to congratulate you! If you have already had surgery then you are on your way to losing weight and getting healthier, and this book will help you on your journey and answer any questions you might have. If you are just considering surgery and are looking for information, this book will help you make the right decision and also understand your options without having to spend countless hours on the Internet getting information from unreliable sources or reviewing medical literature that doesn't make sense. Relax and enjoy the book, I have already done all the research for you! Without any further ado, let's get started!

1. HOW IS OBESITY DEFINED AND HOW DO I DETERMINE IF I SUFFER FROM OBESITY?

Obesity is generally defined based on Body Mass Index, or BMI. This is not a perfect way to define obesity because it does not take into account your lean body mass or body type, but it is the only one available to us at the present time. By definition, BMI is the ratio of your weight (in kilograms) to the square root of your height (in meters):

$$BMI = weight \ (kg)/Height^2 \ (m^2)$$

So you can do the math if you wish or you can go online and find a quick BMI calculator. For example: www.bmi-calculator.net

The reason why you need to know your BMI is to know whether you suffer from obesity and to also find out if you qualify for surgery if you ever decide to have it.

- If your BMI is between 25 and 29.9 you are overweight.
- If your BMI is between 30 and 34.9 you are class I obese, but you will only qualify for a band or gastric balloon, not bypass.

If your BMI is between 35 and 39.9 you are class II obese and you will qualify for surgery as long as you have one other medical condition such as diabetes, high blood pressure or sleep apnea.

- If your BMI is 40 or higher then you are class III obese, also categorized as morbidly obese, and you will qualify even if you are healthy and have no medical issues!

These criteria were put forth by the National Institute of Health (NIH) in 1991 and all the bariatric centers in the US follow these criteria. However, there is growing evidence that even patients with low BMI may benefit from surgery, especially people who have medical conditions like diabetes. Therefore, I wouldn't be surprised if these criteria change in the future and the eligibility based on BMI is lowered. Even now, many centers outside the US are already performing bariatric surgery for patients with lower BMIs. In our center we recently changed our own guidelines and we are now offering bariatric surgery for patients who suffer from uncontrolled diabetes as long as their BMI is 30 or higher.

Many centers have their own eligibility criteria in addition to the BMI criteria. So even if you qualify based on your BMI your surgeon may ask you to undergo additional testing and to get enrolled in a medical weight loss program before performing your surgery. This will be discussed further in the preoperative requirements chapter below.

Now keep in mind that some insurance companies may give you hard time even if you qualify for bariatric surgery based on those BMI criteria. Your health insurance provider may ask for more documentation to show that you have a medical condition and are taking medication for it. But do not get frustrated and do continue to fight for your rights!

2. WHY ARE MORE PEOPLE NOW SUFFERING FROM OBESITY?

Obesity is currently a major problem, it is a pandemic on a bigger scale than the recent COVID-19 pandemic that we all experienced. According to the most recent reports by the Center for Disease Control (CDC), two-thirds of the US population is considered overweight, and one-third is considered obese. Also, 13 percent of the adults in the world are obese and 39 percent are considered overweight.

Even children are not immune, one in every five children and adolescents worldwide are considered overweight. Unfortunately, some groups are affected more than others by the obesity pandemic. For example, African Americans and Hispanics are more affected than others. Obesity is also more common in middle- aged adults between the ages of 40 and 59 compared to other age groups. However, women with college degrees are less affected compared to women without degrees but enough of those boring statistics!. The take home message is this: more and more people are affected, and obesity is becoming the plague of our century!

The reasons behind the obesity epidemic are multi-fold, which means nobody truly knows!

To be more precise, people are not as active as they should be. A study by the United Nations (UN) actually showed that people are physically inactive, which means they are not exercising, as they should. The food industry is also partly to blame due to the high consumption of processed food items and the addition of high fructose corn syrup plus other artificial sweeteners to many of the canned foods that we consume on a daily basis. Not to mention sodas! And yes—even diet sodas are bad for you, but good try! In addition to these factors the technological advances and our current lifestyles are not helping either. Even if you are an active person who likes to read books instead of watching TV or playing video games, if you look into your daily routine very closely you will find that you spend hours every week watching your favorite TV shows. How can you help but watch shows like *House of Card, Money Heist* or *Game of Thrones.*

In addition to this "toxic" environment I mentioned previously, many patients become obese or, more accurately, become afflicted by obesity because of medications or medical problems. For example, medications commonly used to treat depression or psychosis are known for being "obesogenic," meaning they can cause weight gain. At my practice I see many patients who gained weight immediately after they were started on these psychogenic medications. Medical problems like hypothyroidism (underactive thyroid) or Cushing's disease (overactive adrenal gland) can also cause obesity.

In addition, genetics plays a role, having a family history of obesity will put you at a higher risk for becoming obese. Therefore, if you have somebody in the family who suffers from obesity you need to be very careful because that means you are more predisposed to gain weight over time than people without a similar family history. In cases where obesity runs in the patient's family (just like in diabetes or other diseases) the odds are stacked against the patient and the patient has to work very hard, unfortunately, to avoid gaining weight and becoming obese. It is a problem and it is very sad but this is how it is. However, there is hope, as you will find in this book—so keep reading!

3. WHO QUALIFIES FOR BARIATRIC SURGERY?

As mentioned in the previous chapter, according to the NIH guidelines that were published in 1991 any patient whose BMI or body mass index is above 35 and who suffers from at least one obesity-related medical condition like diabetes, elevated blood pressure, or sleep apnea qualifies for a bariatric procedure.

In addition, any patient whose BMI is above 40 whether the patient suffers from a medical condition or not does qualify for a bariatric procedure.

These criteria are old and are in the process of being revised because many recent studies have shown that patients with even lower BMI can benefit from bariatric surgery. However, at this point most bariatric centers in the United States (US) would not operate on any patient whose BMI is less than 30-35. In addition insurance companies that cover bariatric surgery in the US would not cover any procedure unless the patient's BMI is at least 35. Some insurance companies use 40 as their cutoff. Therefore, you need to check with your insurance carrier to make sure that first you have the coverage and to also ask about the specific criteria they are using. Centers outside the US have different inclusion criteria and may operate on patients with BMI less than 35 (if you live in the United States 35 is the magic number!)

If you live outside the US and you are paying for your surgery out of your own pocket, then these BMI cutoffs may not mean much to you. In that case you need to have a discussion with your surgeon based on your BMI, medical condition and risk factors to clearly understand what are the risks and benefits of undergoing bariatric surgery. As previously mentioned, patients with uncontrolled diabetes can now undergo bariatric surgery if their BMI is 30 or more in most of the bariatric centers found in the US (including ours).

4. WHY SHOULD I CONSIDER BARIATRIC SURGERY?

If you suffer from morbid obesity and have a BMI of 35 or more, you owe it to yourself and your family to consider bariatric surgery for many reasons. I will list ten reasons why you should consider bariatric surgery even though there are way more than just ten reasons:

1. Bariatric surgery can lead to significant weight loss, which will often result in improvement or resolution of your medical problems. This should lead to better overall health and result in an extension of your lifespan. Many studies have shown that after bariatric surgery patients live an average of 8 to 10 years longer.

2. Following bariatric surgery, you should become more active and more productive, which could lead to an improvement in the economic status of your family overall. Patients have always told me over the years that following bariatric surgery they became more productive and many of them received promotions at work. I hate to say it but it's true: obese patients are less likely to get a job interview or get hired just because people tend to think of obese patients as lazy and unproductive—only very few people understand that obesity is a disease just like cancer!. Weight bias is a real issue in our society.

Studies have shown that people, even physicians, can be biased and look at patients with obesity very negatively.

3. Bariatric surgery has become a very safe treatment modality so the benefits of undergoing a bariatric procedure far outweigh the risks.

4. Studies have shown that when a parent undergoes surgery the entire family starts losing weight and starts eating in a healthier manner, therefore the entire family may become more active and lose weight.

5. Morbidly obese patients generally suffer from a very poor sex life, including low energy and low sexual desire. However, following bariatric surgery, patients report a significant improvement in their sex lives, including increased interest in and energy for sex.

6. Morbidly obese patients generally have low self-esteem and poor self-confidence and can be shy about speaking in public or appearing in public places. Following bariatric surgery, patients' self-esteem usually improves significantly, and patients usually become more outgoing and more confident. They can live their lives to the fullest. I have heard repeatedly from my patients that following weight loss many felt that they came out of their shell and they were able to experience life like they never could before.

7. Undergoing bariatric surgery is not the easy way out that many people think it is. On the contrary, it is a strong indication that you are taking charge of your life and health and making an effort to turn your life around to be healthier and happier. By undergoing bariatric surgery you are basically acting as a role model

for people around you who suffer from obesity; you are demonstrating that there is a way out if you put your mind to it and if you make the effort to turn your life around.

8. Weight loss surgery will improve your lifestyle and should help prevent the occurrence of health-related complications such as heart attacks, strokes, diabetes, high blood pressure, among others. Accordingly, over the years that follow a bariatric procedure you should find yourself less likely to get sick or to be admitted to a hospital. Many observational studies have shown that the mortality rates of patients who had bariatric surgery do go down, meaning the risk of death from a heart attack or a stroke is reduced.

9. After weight loss you should find yourself more likely to perform activities that you've never thought you could perform, such as riding a bike, taking a ride at an amusement park, hiking, mountain climbing, and yes, even skydiving.

10. Losing weight will improve your emotional and mental well-being and your sense of achievement and satisfaction.

5. WHAT ARE THE BARIATRIC PROCEDURES AVAILABLE TO ME?

There are many bariatric procedures that are currently being performed. Some of these may be more popular than others depending on where you live and also depending on your surgeon's preference. These options include:

1. Sleeve gastrectomy (SG)

2. Adjustable gastric banding (AGB)

3. Gastric bypass (RYGB)

4. Intra-gastric balloon (GB)

5. Biliopancreatic diversion (BPD/DS) and Single Anastomosis Duodenal Ileostomy (SADI)

6. Mini/gastric bypass (MGB)

The two most commonly performed procedures in the US are the sleeve gastrectomy (SG) and the gastric bypass (RYGB.) Gastric banding (AGB) is falling out of favor because of less favorable long-term outcomes such as poor weight loss and complications. Biliopancreatic diversion (BPD/DS) is a relatively high-risk procedure and usually reserved for patients with extremely high BMI. Less than 1 percent of all the procedures performed in the US are (BPD/DS). However, a new modified and simpler version of the BPD/DS called SADI is now more commonly performed and is becoming more popular. The intra-gastric balloon procedure was recently approved by the Food and Drug Administration and is currently being performed in the US for patients with a BMI of between 30 and 40 who suffer from at least one obesity-associated medical condition. However, GB is not covered by insurance and can cost up to $9,000. Mini-gastric bypass (MGB) is rarely offered in the US but is common in Europe, Latin America, and the Middle East.

We have no solid scientific evidence to recommend one bariatric procedure over another so the choice of the best bariatric procedure for any particular patient depends on the patient factors such as their expectations and their past surgical and medical history, in addition to the expertise of the local surgeons and institutions.

Every procedure has its own advantages and disadvantages. Below is a brief description of each procedure with a list of advantages and disadvantages, including potential complications. The following applies to the laparoscopic approach because that is the approach that most surgeons use these days, including Dr. E.

1. Sleeve gastrectomy

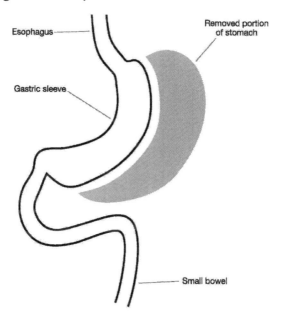

The sleeve gastrectomy is a restrictive procedure that causes weight loss by reducing the size of the stomach to initially hold about 150–300ml. During the procedure, 75-85 percent of the stomach is surgically removed.

After the procedure the stomach will look like a tube or a banana. The staples used to transect your stomach will keep your new stomach closed. Because part of your stomach is removed the procedure is not reversible.

There is no re-routing of your intestine or adjustment needed following sleeve gastrectomy. The procedure is performed laparoscopically using small incisions. The procedure takes around 45 to 60 minutes to perform and is very safe and effective. Weight loss following sleeve gastrectomy is usually 60–65 percent of the excess weight. Hospital stay following sleeve gastrectomy is usually 1 to 2 days.

To qualify for a sleeve gastrectomy, you should fall into one of those two categories:

1. BMI of 40 or higher
2. BMI of 35 or higher, with at least one obesity-associated medical condition like high blood pressure, sleep apnea or diabetes.

Advantages:

1. Excellent safety profile
2. Incidence of post-operative complications is between 1 and 5 percent
3. Short term results similar to gastric bypass
4. Malabsorption is minimal
5. No dumping
6. Short hospital stay
7. No hernias or marginal ulcers

Disadvantages:

1. Vitamin deficiencies can occur when patients do not take their daily vitamins.
2. Heartburn, bloating, and epigastric pain can occur after sleeve gastrectomy.
3. Long-term weight loss is less than gastric bypass.
4. Hair loss can occur but is usually self-limited and can be prevented by taking biotin and protein supplements.
5. Gallstones happen in only 5 percent of patients following a sleeve gastrectomy. If you develop pain because

of gallstones you may need to have your gallbladder removed.

2. Gastric bypass

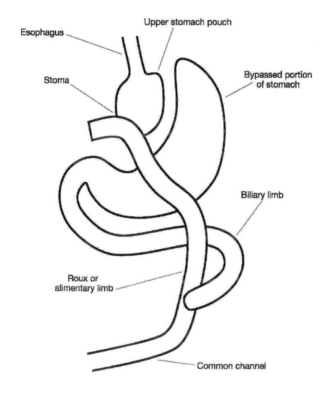

Laparoscopic gastric bypass is a restrictive weight loss procedure, which is performed by making five small incisions in the patient's abdominal wall using small instruments and a camera. The procedure takes around 1 to 1.5 hours to perform. A small pouch (30-50 ml), roughly the size of an egg, is created from the upper portion of the stomach using a stapling device and then a portion of the small intestine is cut and connected to the pouch. After the procedure, you will feel full more quickly. This reduces the amount of food you can eat at one time. Bypassing a portion of the intestine will also reduce the amount of food and nutrients that is absorbed.

The weight loss achieved after a gastric bypass is secondary to the restriction created by the small pouch and the malabsorption that results from the bypassed portion of the small intestine. In addition, the procedure has profound metabolic and hormonal effects, which lead to weight loss, appetite suppression, and resolution of diabetes. The amount of excess weight loss in the first 12 months is around 70 to 85 percent. The hospital stay is usually 1 to 2 days.

In order to know whether you qualify for a gastric bypass you need to know your BMI.

To qualify for a gastric bypass, you should fall into one of those two categories:

1. BMI of 40 or higher

2. BMI of 35 or higher, with at least one obesity-associated medical condition like high blood pressure, sleep apnea, or diabetes.

Advantages:

1. Excellent safety profile

2. Incidence of post-operative complications less than 5 percent

3. Excellent long term results

4. Weight loss after a gastric bypass exceeds weight loss by other bariatric procedures like sleeve gastrectomy and gastric banding

5. Minimal side effects

6. Short hospital stay

7. Reversible

Disadvantages:

1. Vitamin deficiencies can occur when patients do not take their daily vitamins.

2. Dumping syndrome occurs when food enters the small intestine too quickly resulting in nausea, feeling shaky, and diarrhea.

3. Hair loss can occur, but is usually self-limited and can be prevented by taking biotin and protein supplements.

4. Gallstones form in only 10 percent of patients following a gastric bypass. If you develop pain because of the gallstones you may need to have your gallbladder removed.

5. Marginal ulcers can occur especially in smokers and patients who are not taking proton pump inhibitors.

6. Internal hernias can develop after weight loss and may require surgical correction.

3. Adjustable gastric banding

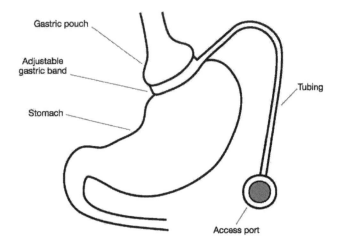

Gastric pouch

Adjustable
gastric band

Tubing

Stomach

Access port

A silicone band is placed around the upper portion of the stomach forming a small pouch and a small opening for food to pass through. This small pouch restricts the amount of food one is able to eat.

The band is adjusted through the injection of saline solution into a port placed under the skin of the abdominal wall. Adjustments are performed 6 weeks following surgery. Weight loss averages 1 to 2 pounds per week.

Gastric banding is usually effective in young, healthy, and active patients who have low BMIs. Patients with high BMIs and co-morbidities are encouraged to undergo a bypass or a sleeve gastrectomy instead of an adjustable gastric banding.

Laparoscopic banding is a very low-risk procedure that can be performed as an outpatient.

To qualify for gastric banding, you should fall into one of those two categories:

1. BMI of 40 or higher

2. BMI of 30 or higher, with at least one obesity associated medical condition like high blood pressure, sleep apnea or diabetes.

Advantages:

1. Excellent safety profile

2. Short procedure that can be performed as a same-day surgery

3. No stapling of the stomach or small intestine

4. No marginal ulcers or hernias

5. No dumping syndrome

6. No malabsorption

Disadvantages:

1. Can result in heartburn or nausea and vomiting

2. Weight loss is lower than other bariatric procedures

3. Can result in slippage, erosion, or pouch dilatation over time.

4. Requires repeated adjustments

4. Intra-gastric balloon

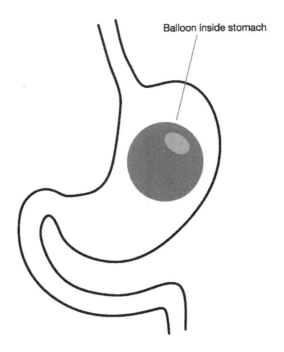

Balloon inside stomach

The two recently FDA-approved balloons currently on the market are:

- Orbera ® balloon
- Reshape ® balloon

Both balloons are offered for patients who have a BMI of 30–40 with at least one medical condition. The balloon is placed endoscopically, meaning non-surgically. It usually takes 30 minutes for placement and most people go home the same day. The balloon is usually placed and then left in place for 6 months before being removed (the new Orbera ® 365 can be left in place for 12 months). After the removal of the balloon you will continue to receive counseling for up to one year. Also, both companies provide online support to track your progress.

A new balloon called Elipse® by allurion is currently available outside the US. It's a balloon that comes in a capsule form that is connected to a thin tube. Once the capsule is swallowed and is in the stomach, your doctor will use the tube to fill the capsule with liquid. No need for anesthesia or endoscopy. After 4 months the balloon deflates on its own and comes out. As previously mentioned this is not FDA approved and is not available in the US.

Advantages:

1. Non-surgical

2. Removable and non-permanent

3. Minimal to no pain or discomfort

4. Patients are discharged the same day

5. Suppresses the appetite and results in quick satiety when eating

Disadvantages:

1. Weight loss is much less compared to other procedures

2. Weight gain after balloon removal is a possibility

3. Results in nausea and vomiting in the first few weeks after insertion

4. Not covered by insurance and can be expensive

5. Biliopancreatic diversion with duodenal switch (BPD/DS)

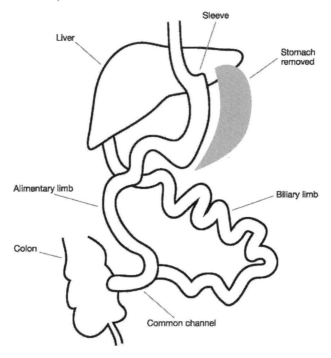

This procedure is an advanced weight loss procedure that is not commonly performed by bariatric surgeons because it is a high-risk surgery that can lead to serious health issues. However, in experienced hands the procedure is as safe as a gastric bypass. It is usually offered for super-obese patients—those with a BMI of 50 or higher.

The procedure is basically a combination of the gastric bypass and the sleeve gastrectomy. There are two bilio-pancreatic diversion surgeries: with and without duodenal switch. During the procedure the stomach is reduced in size just like in a sleeve gastrectomy and then the intestine is bypassed and connected to the duodenum (duodenal switch) or the stomach (no duodenal switch.)

The procedure involving the duodenal switch is more common and is the one shown here.

The procedure takes around 3 hours and is usually offered for patients with high BMIs, uncontrolled diabetes, or hypercholesterolemia. The procedure is performed laparoscopically using small incisions. Weight loss is similar to or slightly higher than gastric bypass and the hospital stay following the procedure is usually 1 to 2 days.

In order to know whether you qualify for a BPD you need to know your BMI.

To qualify for a BPD you should fall into one of those two categories:

1. BMI of 40 or higher

2. BMI of 35 or higher, with at least one obesity-associated medical condition like high blood pressure, sleep apnea, or diabetes.

Advantages:

1. Excellent short- and long-term weight loss results that exceed other bariatric procedures.

2. Rate of resolution of co-morbidities following surgery is higher than other bariatric procedures.

3. Very effective for super obese patients (BMI of 50 or higher.)

4. Short hospital stay.

5. No marginal ulcers (BPD with duodenal switch.)

Disadvantages:

1. Higher incidence of vitamin deficiencies compared to gastric bypass especially when patients are not taking their daily vitamins.

2. Heartburn can occur after BPD with duodenal switch.

3. This procedure can result in frequent loose stools (diarrhea), which usually improves over time.

4. Protein malnutrition occurs in a small number of cases.

5. Abdominal bloating and malodorous gas.

The Single Anastomosis Duodenal Ileostomy (SADI) sometimes called SIPS or loop duodenal switch is a modification of the original BPD which was recently endorsed by the American Society of Metabolic and Bariatric Surgery (ASMBS). SADI entails the performance of a sleeve in addition to a simple connection between the bowel and duodenum. This procedure is becoming popular because of its ease and good outcomes especially in patients who underwent a sleeve gastrectomy previously but are gaining weight.

6. Mini-gastric Bypass

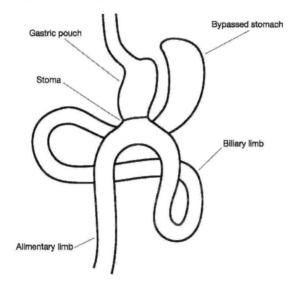

Laparoscopic mini/gastric bypass is a restrictive weight loss procedure just like the regular gastric bypass but less invasive because there is no rerouting of the bowel. It is also performed by making multiple small incisions in the patient's abdominal wall and by using small instruments and a camera. The procedure takes a little less time than the gastric bypass to perform, usually around 1 hour.

A small pouch (30–50 ml) is also created from the upper portion of the stomach using a stapling device and then the small intestine is connected to the pouch directly without re-routing. After the procedure, you will feel full more quickly than when your stomach was its original size. This reduces the amount of food you can eat at one time. Even though we are not bypassing any segment of the bowel there is still malabsorption.

The weight loss achieved after a mini-gastric bypass is secondary to the restriction created by the small pouch and the malabsorption and is, for the most part, very similar to the gastric bypass. The amount of excess weight loss in the first 12 months is around 70 to 75 percent. Hospital stay is usually 1 to 2 days.

In order to know whether you qualify for a mini-gastric bypass you need to know your BMI.

1. BMI of 40 or higher

2. BMI of 35 or higher, with at least one obesity-associated medical condition like high blood pressure, sleep apnea, or diabetes.

Keep in mind that the mini-gastric bypass is more common in countries other than the US and in those countries the BMI criteria are less stringent.

Advantages:

1. Excellent safety profile

2. Incidence of post-operative complications is less than 5 percent

3. Excellent long-term results

4. Weight loss after a mini-gastric bypass is similar to weight loss after a gastric bypass

5. Minimal side effects

6. Short hospital stay

7. Reversible and less invasive than a gastric bypass

8. No internal hernias

Disadvantages:

1. Vitamin deficiencies can occur when patients are not taking their vitamins.

2. Dumping syndrome can occur when food enters the small intestine too quickly resulting in nausea, shaky feeling, and diarrhea.

3. Hair loss can occur but is usually self-limited and can be prevented by taking biotin and protein supplements.

4. Marginal ulcers can occur especially in smokers and patients who are not taking proton pump inhibitors.

Before you meet with your surgeon make sure you review the advantages and disadvantages of each procedure in order to be able to discuss with your doctor which procedure is more appropriate for you. Your surgeon should discuss all these options with you during the consultation, but it will be very helpful if you do some research ahead of time. I always tell my patients during the information seminars to review our website www. slhn.org/bariatrics and do some research ahead of time and prepare a list of questions before they come and see me in the office.

6. HOW SHOULD I CHOOSE MY SURGEON?

It is very important for anyone considering bariatric surgery to do some research prior to choosing a hospital or a surgeon.

Bariatric surgery is very different than gallbladder surgery or hernia surgery. Firstly, bariatric surgery is technically difficult and complicated so the surgeon performing bariatric surgery should be especially trained to be able to perform these kinds of surgeries safely. Secondly, the surgeon should be experienced enough in managing bariatric complications in case you develop a complication or an adverse event.

In the US, there are two types of surgeons who perform bariatric surgery: the first group are general surgeons who have completed general surgery training and then developed an interest in performing bariatric or weight loss surgery; the second group are general surgeons who have completed a fellowship (i.e. additional training in bariatric surgery after the completion of general surgery training). In general, fellowship-trained surgeons are more experienced in performing these kinds of surgeries but many general surgeons also have a vast experience in bariatric surgery so you need to do your research before choosing your surgeon. If you have a choice I would recommend you choose a fellowship-trained surgeon—as long as he or she has a good reputation of course!

The American Society of Metabolic and Bariatric Surgery has a website that lists all available bariatric surgeons in your area. You can visit www.asmbs.org, go to "patients" and click "find a provider."

This Website lists all the surgeons who perform bariatric surgery in your area but does not tell you how qualified the surgeons are. It is your job to research each surgeon by checking their Website and their credentials.

Another useful Website is the American College of Surgeons (ACS) Website (www. facs.org). Go to "find a surgeon" and under the specialty drop down menu you can select "general surgery" for the Website to give you a list of all the general surgeons in your area. You can then pick surgeons who perform bariatric surgery and also review their credentials. Again, the ACS website does not give you any information about each surgeon's outcome history and experience but you can quickly review their education, training, and areas of expertise to be able to decide for yourself based on what I have mentioned above.

When you meet your surgeon for the first time make sure you ask the following ten questions:

1. What kind of training did you undergo and what are your credentials to perform bariatric surgery?

2. Is there coverage after hours by another bariatric surgeon to handle emergencies?

3. What is your complication rate?

4. What is the outcome of bariatric patients in your practice?

5. What kind of postoperative support is available in your center or practice?

6. Is dietary counseling and social support by a licensed social worker or psychologist available at the practice?

7. How frequently will I be seen after surgery?

8. Who will be handling my questions or phone calls in the future if I have questions or concerns?

9. Do I have access to support groups following surgery?

10. Is there an insurance specialist at the practice to help me navigate all the insurance hurdles?

After asking these 10 very important questions you will have a very good idea whether your surgeon is truly qualified to perform your surgery and whether the program your surgeon has in place is a comprehensive and multidisciplinary program.

7. WHICH IS BETTER FOR ME, SLEEVE GASTRECTOMY OR GASTRIC BYPASS?

This question comes up regularly during consultations and information seminars. The question is a very important question but not a straightforward one. In this chapter, I will quickly review the available medical literature in simple terms and tell you about my experience after performing both procedures for more than 10 years. Even though laparoscopic sleeve gastrectomy is a very safe and effective procedure and is routinely offered by most surgeons, patients and health care providers counseling patients on weight loss procedures need to be aware of a few differences between sleeve gastrectomy and gastric bypass.

First, both procedures when performed in accredited centers by experienced surgeons are safe and effective. The claim that sleeve is safer than bypass does not stand up when the literature is carefully reviewed. The overall complication rate of both procedures is less than 5 percent and the major complication rate such as leaking or bleeding is around 1 percent. However, readmission rates are usually higher with bypass patients because of dehydration and early nausea and vomiting after the procedure.

Second, weight loss achieved after a gastric bypass is on average 15–25 percent higher than the weight loss achieved following a sleeve. On average, gastric bypass patients achieve

75–85 percent excess weight loss at 12 months compared to 60–65 percent with a sleeve gastrectomy. In addition, after the first 12 months, sleeve patients have a higher incidence of weight regain. I always emphasize that long-term success is patient driven and that compliance plays a major role in the overall success. However, our data, and data from other centers, has shown that recidivism, or weight regain, is slightly higher in sleeve patients compared to bypass patients especially after the first or second year.

The reasons why patients gain weight following sleeve is multifactorial and may be related to the dilatation of the stomach over time or to the loss of appetite suppression the patients enjoy initially after a sleeve gastrectomy. On the other hand, patients whose BMI is less than 40 and undergo a sleeve gastrectomy do as well as bypass patients in terms of weight loss so BMI needs to be taken into account as well as patient preference.

The sleeve gastrectomy is a well-established procedure with good short- and intermediate-term results. In addition, it does not involve any suturing or stapling of the small bowel as previously mentioned and thus it has become a very popular procedure. Sleeve gastrectomy is currently the most commonly performed procedure in the US and around the world and it continues to gain momentum. The gastric band has fallen out of favor because of the high reoperation rate, long-term complications, and poor weight loss. The sleeve gastrectomy has basically replaced the gastric band in most centers in the US.

Sleeve gastrectomy is a relatively simple procedure but has to be performed by a highly skilled bariatric surgeon for it to work, if this is not the case the patient may not experience any weight loss. Additionally, if not performed properly it can result in severe reflux, abdominal pain, chronic nausea and vomiting.

In certain cases, we have even seen sleeve "migration" into the chest which again can cause heartburn, chest pain, nausea and vomiting. The sleeve gastrectomy is also a relatively new procedure, which means long- term results are not available so far. Even though we have seen some reports showing good long-term excess weight loss results compared to the gastric bypass, whether the sleeve is comparable to the gastric bypass or not beyond the first 2 to 5 years is still open for debate.

I have seen very good short-term results when comparing my sleeve patients to the gastric bypass patients, but long-term gastric bypass patients achieved on average 15 percent more excess weight at the 1-year mark.

The gastric bypass remains, at this time, the gold standard of all bariatric surgeries against which all the other procedures are usually compared including the sleeve gastrectomy. Gastric bypass has excellent short- and long-term results and when performed by an experienced surgeon is as safe as gallbladder surgery.

So, after saying all of this, which is better?

The decision on whether to perform a bypass or a sleeve for a specific patient has to be individualized based on age, BMI and patient preference. Also, health issues like diabetes and heartburn have to be taken into account. The patient ultimately makes the decision after being well informed of all the advantages and disadvantages of each procedure. As a useful guide I will provide a list of certain conditions which make one procedure preferable over the other, but you should have this discussion with your surgeon, he or she knows your medical condition better than anybody else.

In the following cases, a gastric bypass is preferable:

- High BMI
- History of heartburn
- Young patients
- Presence of a hiatal or a paraoesophageal hernia
- Presence of diabetes or pre-diabetes
- Presence of Barrett's esophagus

In the following cases, a sleeve gastrectomy is preferable:

- Presence of gastric polyps (depending on the type of polyps)
- Presence of inflammatory bowel disease
- History of open surgeries or incisional hernias repaired with synthetic mesh (plastic)
- Concern about compliance with vitamin intake
- Need for long term treatment with blood thinners like anti-platelets or need for recurrent use of NSAID

8. WHAT IS REVISION SURGERY AND WILL I NEED A REVISION AFTER MY PROCEDURE?

As mentioned previously, bariatric surgery has a high success rate and it is very unusual for bariatric patients to develop complications as long as the surgery is performed in an accredited center by an experienced surgeon. Saying that, and given that around 250,000 bariatric procedures are performed every year in the US, bariatric surgeons do, in general, encounter patients who develop complications following surgery and are in dire need for revisional surgery. In addition, weight regain after surgery can be an issue—hence my emphasis on compliance and the need to be committed to the lifelong lifestyle change that is needed after surgery as discussed previously—and may also require revisional surgery.

So, what is revisional surgery? Revisional surgery is simply any bariatric surgery that is performed on a patient who has already had bariatric surgery in the past. Revisional surgery includes a large variety of surgical procedures that are anything but similar. To simplify the issue and for the sake of the discussion I will divide the procedures into two types:

1. Revisional surgery to correct anatomical issues: this includes all surgeries performed to correct an anatomi-

cal problem like a stricture, ulcer, obstruction, dilated pouch, fistula, etc.

2. Revisional surgery for weight regain (or recidivism): this includes conversions performed to convert one type of procedure into a different type to address a specific issue or to cause more weight loss. Examples of conversions include band conversion to bypass or sleeve conversion to a bypass or even band to sleeve, etc.

You don't need to know the different types of surgery out there and what they are called, the only thing you do need to know is that in the unfortunate case that you develop a problem or fail to lose the expected weight, there is help available and you should seek the expertise of a bariatric surgeon who is experienced in those kind of procedures in order to assist you.

For the sake of illustration I will list some current issues facing patients who have had bariatric surgery: The two main issues are surgical complications and weight regain!

Weight regain: Studies suggest that 10 to 30 percent of patients are unable to meet their target weight or they regain significant weight following bariatric surgery.

Surgical complications: Although uncommon, bariatric surgery patients can develop a number of surgical complications following surgery like fistulas, heartburn and regurgitation, marginal ulcers, obstruction or blockage or even leak.

Revisional procedures are usually performed laparoscopically but sometimes they have to be done in an open fashion (by making a large incision in your abdomen) especially when dealing with complications. Luckily, now that we are using robotic surgery to perform these cases, we have much better instruments and better visualization so it is uncommon to have to do an open surgery to address these issues.

I personally continue to perform all my revisional surgeries either laparoscopically or, even better, with the assistance of the robot, this has improved the outcomes of those complicated procedures significantly. In certain cases complications can be addressed and treated endoscopically (by using an endoscope without the need for surgery) but this is usually done only in specialized centers so always ask your surgeon if there is any minimally invasive option to treat your problem without undergoing surgery. For example, certain centers, including ours, can address a dilated pouch or stoma endoscopically by suturing it from the inside without the need for surgery using special suturing instruments.

For similar non-invasive procedures you may have to be referred to an expert in endoscopy to address your problem. Your surgeon will be able to help you decide which approach is more appropriate for your specific condition. Always ask about the options available to you and do your research before making a decision.

Examples of revisional procedures are:

- Correction of dilated gastric pouch or dilated gastric stoma (opening)

- Conversion of sleeve gastrectomy to gastric bypass for weight regain or heartburn

- Conversion of sleeve gastrectomy to biliopancreatic diversion for weight regain or for the purpose of additional weight loss

- Correction of stoma (opening) stricture in a gastric bypass

- Correction of chronic obstruction (blockage) in gastric bypass
- Correction of large hiatal hernias in bariatric patients
- Correction of an esophageal disorder
- Correction of gastric fistulas (abnormal connection between your pouch and old stomach) following gastric bypass surgery
- Correction of chronic marginal ulcers following gastric bypass surgery
- Conversion of vertical banded gastroplasty (VBG) to a gastric bypass

Keep in mind that these procedures are not to be taken lightly. These can be very difficult procedures, so do your research and pick an experienced surgeon to address your issue. The complication rates after these procedures are usually higher than your average everyday bariatric procedure so be mentally prepared for that and expect to be in hospital for a few extra days. However, saying that, because of the more recent adoption of robotic surgery at our center and other centers, we have seen those technically challenging cases performed very safely and patients discharged in a day or two at the most.

Patients do have to undergo some tests before surgery, just like with any kind of surgery. In addition to these tests, patients undergoing a conversion because of poor weight loss may have to complete a few months of physician-supervised diet programs before they qualify for an alternative weight loss procedure.

Insurance coverage for these procedures can also be an issue. If the revision surgery is performed to correct an anatomical problem or to address a complication then coverage is usually not a problem because this is considered "medically necessary" by most insurance companies. Even then the documentation needs to be really good and your surgeon should be willing to talk in person to the medical director of your insurance company if need be in order to explain the nature of your medical situation. The biggest problem we encounter is when we try to perform a conversion from one weight loss procedure to another because of poor weight loss or weight regain.

In those situations, unfortunately, patients are usually denied coverage and the argument usually made by insurance carriers (and it's always the same argument) is that a patient only gets one chance to lose weight with surgery and that patient blew his or her chance, they were not compliant as evidenced by the lack of weight loss, and therefore that person would not be given another chance. These decisions are usually made by policymakers who do not have a good understanding of why bariatric patients gain weight over time and of the chronic nature of obesity (I always say that obesity is a chronic disease just like cancer and it can always come back). Insurance companies will not deny a patient medical coverage if the patient had cancer, was treated for it and then developed recurrence, but when it comes to obesity they tend to blame the patient and not the disease.

If this happens to you, your best bet is to file an appeal but this has to be coordinated closely with your surgeon and the supporting office staff. What needs to be done in these situations is to build a strong case to show that despite your best efforts and despite being compliant you failed to lose the weight you expected to lose because of the nature of the procedure. We have this problem now with band and sleeve patients who fail to lose any weight.

Most weight loss centers that deal with revision patients on a regular basis will enroll you in a structured physician-supervised weight loss program to monitor your commitment and compliance prior to performing a revisional bariatric procedure. After the completion of such a program your surgeon will decide, based on the input of the entire team, whether you will benefit from a revision or not and whether you truly qualify for a second procedure based on your BMI, medical conditions, and your commitment. The documentation obtained throughout that time period can then be used to get you approved by your insurance provider.

9. WHY DO I HAVE TO COMPLETE A PHYSICIAN-SUPERVISED MEDICAL DIET BEFORE SURGERY?

Some insurance carriers require bariatric patients to complete 3 to 6 months of physician-supervised weight loss. This includes either monthly documentation of weights in a physician's office or physician encounters with documentation of weight loss. More recently some insurance carriers have even required 12 months of physician supervised medical encounters.

This requirement is usually applied without any regard to the patient's previous attempts at weight loss. Commercially available programs such as Weight Watchers or Jenny Craig, which are used by a lot of our patients are not usually taken into account by insurance companies. In addition, a lot of the bariatric patients have severe co-morbid conditions or obesity-related health conditions that can be life-threatening. Waiting for up to 6 or 12 months before performing bariatric surgery can only worsen these conditions.

This behavior on the part of insurance carriers is frustrating to patients and is not financially sustainable. Patients who have to comply with these terms complain to me and my staff about this all the time! Most of the patients have to take time off work to go to the physician's office for a weight check. In addition, when insurance carriers require a physician encounter, the visits may not be covered by insurance and the patients sometimes have to pay out of their pocket. Some patients are even penalized if they miss an appointment and have to start the process all over again.

Following many inquiries by hospitals, surgeons, and patients, the American Society of Metabolic and Bariatric Surgery (ASMBS) put out a statement saying that there are no evidence-based reports that document the benefit of, or the need for, a 3 or 6 months preoperative dietary weight loss program before bariatric surgery. According to the ASMBS, this mandated preoperative weight loss can lead to patient inconvenience, frustration, healthcare costs, and lost income due to the requirement for repeated physician visits that are not covered by health insurance. The ASMBS also stated that it is the position of the ASMBS that the requirement for documentation of prolonged preoperative diet efforts before health insurance carrier approval of bariatric surgery services is inappropriate, capricious, and counter-productive given the complete absence of a reasonable level of medical evidence to support this practice.

The ASMBS has pointed out that "policies such as these, that delay, impede or otherwise interfere with life-saving and cost-effective treatment, as have been proven to be true for bariatric surgery in the treatment of morbid obesity, are unacceptable without supporting evidence." Many surgeons have studied the issue and found that insurance-mandated weight loss programs result in a significant delay in receiving surgical treatment and result in no significant preoperative or postoperative weight loss.

On the other hand, we usually ask our patients to lose 5–10 percent of their actual weight prior to bariatric surgery. We, like many other centers, support this diet-induced weight loss prior to surgery in order to decrease liver size and the amount of visceral or intra-abdominal fat. This weight loss usually makes the laparoscopic or robotic approach technically easier and much safer.

In addition, some studies have shown that preoperative weight loss results in shorter hospital stays, faster recovery, less blood loss, and improved postoperative weight loss, at least in the short term following bariatric surgery. Even though the ASMBS did not make specific recommendations regarding this preoperative weight loss, it stated that individual surgeons and programs should be free to recommend preoperative weight loss based on the specific needs and circumstances of the patients.

At our center we are big advocates of patient safety and good patient outcomes, we therefore believe that a small amount of preoperative weight loss (not 3–6 months physician-supervised medical weight loss) is necessary prior to bariatric surgery. Preoperative weight loss has therefore become a requirement of our program. We have also recently instituted a new "enhanced recovery" protocol that helps reduce postoperative pain and avoid low blood sugars immediately before and after surgery.

Ask your surgeon if preoperative weight loss is required before you undergo surgery.

10. WHAT SHOULD I LOOK FOR IN A BARIATRIC PROGRAM?

Choosing a good bariatric program is of paramount importance for your success at the time of surgery and also afterwards. We talked in a previous chapter about the importance of doing some research ahead of time and choosing a well-qualified surgeon. The choice of the weight loss program is as important if not more important than choosing a surgeon.

Primarily, most bariatric patients have many medical problems like diabetes, high blood pressure, sleep apnea, and others, so it is really very important to choose a program that has a process in place to order all the appropriate tests preoperatively to make sure your medical issues are appropriately addressed and managed. Also, the program you choose should have on-site dietitians and certified social workers or psychologists.

Dietitians play a major role in any bariatric program. Dietitians meet with patients before surgery to go over the postoperative diet and also counsel patients on all the healthy eating habits. For example, dietitians usually teach patients about food pyramids, portion control, and also reading food labels. After surgery, dietitians continue to see patients on a regular basis to make sure that they are following the instructions and taking their vitamins. Dietitians also help people struggling with weight loss after surgery.

Social workers and psychologists are also very important in bariatric programs to manage many of the social challenges that bariatric patients face. Social workers and psychologists also address the many psychiatric diseases that bariatric patients suffer from, such as anxiety, depression, obsessive compulsive disorder, and schizophrenia. They also manage drug and alcohol addiction. Many bariatric patients face numerous challenges following their surgery, these can include low self-esteem, interpersonal problems, addiction transfer, and even suicidal ideation; having a social worker or a psychologist on staff in the bariatric program is truly very valuable for postoperative support.

Many weight loss programs also have bariatricians or medical weight loss specialists who can help you achieve some weight loss preoperatively before undergoing surgery which can make the surgery safer and can also assist your surgeon in optimizing your medical conditions before surgery and even afterwards. The presence of a medical weight loss program can also help you maintain your weight loss after achieving your goal following surgery. Again, although not truly necessary in a bariatric program, the presence of a medical weight loss program can be very helpful. The discipline of bariatric surgery is rapidly changing and now more than ever surgeons and obesity specialists (bariatricians) are working closely to manage obesity using a multidisciplinary approach that combines surgery, lifestyle intervention and even medications.

Many surgeons, including myself, have sought additional training in obesity medicine by the American Board of Obesity Medicine (ABOM), in order to be able to better manage their patients using non-surgical means like lifestyle intervention and adjuvant pharmacotherapy in addition to bariatric surgery.

11. WHAT SHOULD I DO IF I DON'T LOSE WEIGHT AFTER BARIATRIC SURGERY?

Weight loss surgery is very efficacious and the success rate after surgery is very high (nothing is 100 percent but the success rate after bariatric surgery can be up to 90 percent.) As we will discuss in a separate chapter the success after weight loss surgery can be defined based on either the cure from the medical conditions that patients suffer from or the amount of weight loss achieved after surgery.

The issue of success and weight loss is a very sensitive one which is why I do not personally like to give my patients goal weights (even though the patients always ask me about their goal weights). When patients come to the office and ask me whether I believe they are successful or not we usually discuss how surgery changed their lives on all levels before concluding whether they have succeeded or not in achieving their goals.

Saying that, the widely accepted definition of success in the medical literature is any weight loss higher than 50 percent of Excess Weight Loss (EWL). For example, if a patient is 100 pounds overweight, he or she needs to lose at least 50 pounds to be considered successful. However, keep in mind that we don't only operate on patients because they are obese, we do operate on a lot of patients because of their illnesses and people who are cured of those illnesses following weight loss surgery in my opinion are very successful irrespective of the amount of weight they lost. That is why when you think about success after surgery you need to remember the reasons behind your decision to have the surgery in the first place. If you are diabetic and you had a gastric bypass because of that and if you stopped taking your diabetic medications (or even insulin) after your surgery because your blood sugar readings are now within normal limits then you are very successful irrespective of how much weight you have lost!

Overall, if we look at the issue of weight loss alone, 10 percent of patients fail to lose weight after surgery. The reasons why people fail to lose weight after surgery are very complicated and we don't really know how to predict who will or who won't lose weight.

Let me try to simplify the issue and explain it further.

There are many factors that can lead to poor or no weight loss after bariatric surgery. Those factors can be divided into patient-specific factors, anatomical factors, and procedure-specific factors. In addition, there are many physiologic changes that happen following bariatric surgery, such as the changes in the level of hormones that we mentioned previously, which can cause weight gain after an initial phase of successful weight loss. Again, fortunately for our patients, the percentage of patients who fail to lose weight following bariatric surgery in a comprehensive center with a proven track record of successful operative outcome and good postoperative patient support system is very low. Postoperative support is really very important as I mention in this book many, many times.

Patient-specific factors include age, race, gender, initial BMI, and patient compliance. For example, elderly patients do lose on average less weight compared to younger patients. Patients with higher initial BMI do lose more pounds but less in terms of percent EWL compared to patients with lower BMI. Compliance also plays a major role in the success rate of patients. If we look, for example, to compliance based on the number of missed visits before and after surgery we find that patients who are not compliant and miss their appointments lose less weight compared to their peers. Please don't miss any appointments!

Anatomical factors that can lead to weight regain or poor weight loss include a large gastric pouch, a large hiatal hernia, a large gastrojejunostomy opening or "stoma," and also a gastro-gastric fistula which is an abnormal connection between the newly created gastric pouch and the old stomach. All those anatomical issues can lead to weight gain and also can result in symptoms like pain, heartburn, regurgitation, and pain upon eating (dysphagia).

Procedure-related factors depend on the weight loss procedure that was chosen initially. Failure rates vary depending on the nature of the procedure that was performed initially. For example, adjustable gastric band placement has a higher failure rate compared to gastric bypass or sleeve gastrectomy. Much higher than the 10 percent I mentioned previously. In addition, malabsorptive procedures like the gastric bypass or the biliopancreatic diversion usually result in higher weight loss compared to purely restrictive procedures like gastric banding or sleeve gastrectomy.

So, what should you do if you stop losing weight or you start regaining weight?

Talk to your doctor.

Bariatric surgeons are aware of the reasons behind weight loss failure and will order a battery of tests to make sure you don't have any of the above mentioned problems that can explain the lack of weight loss or weight regain. Those tests usually include blood work, radiographic studies or even endoscopy. After reviewing those tests your surgeon will discuss your options with you. You may or may not need an operation to correct the problem and make you lose weight again—please refer to the chapter on revision surgery below. In most cases, you will be able to achieve your goals with just counseling and support and some extra effort on your behalf!

12. DO I NEED TO EXERCISE AFTER BARIATRIC SURGERY?

We all know that it is extremely difficult for patients with obesity to exercise on a regular basis because of the physical challenges they have to deal with. Many studies have shown that patients who suffer from obesity have physical challenges related to joint pain and poor functional status and therefore exercising, even though highly desirable, can be very challenging and sometimes near impossible. Try to walk few steps with 100- or 200-pound sandbags on your back and you will know exactly what I mean by that!

Following bariatric surgery, patients lose a significant amount of their excess weight. This usually results in an improvement in their physical ability to exercise. For that reason, we encourage all bariatric patients to start exercising a few weeks after surgery.

We all know that exercising is beneficial. Physicians always encourage their patients to exercise to decrease their risks of developing cardiovascular accidents like stroke and heart attack. For bariatric patients, physical exercise is not only beneficial but also extremely important for the patients to achieve the maximum weight loss after surgery and also to keep the weight off.

Studies have shown that people who exercise after bariatric surgery can achieve more weight loss compared to patients who do not exercise. In addition, exercise will increase your metabolism, which prevents weight gain over time. We also know that the patient's chances of curing their diseases like high blood pressure and diabetes improve when they exercise following surgery. Exercise also helps patients maintain their lean body mass. This will make you feel healthy and also look good! The current recommendation is to exercise around 200–300 minutes per week following surgery. This may sound too much but it is not as long as you start slow and build up your endurance over time.

After the first 12 to 18 months following bariatric surgery patients usually stop losing weight and they hit what we call a "plateau." After that, patients tend to gain some weight back, around 5 or 10 percent of their initial weight. To prevent any further weight gain and to maintain the weight loss it is very important for the patient to exercise on a regular basis to increase what we call "energy expenditure," which is just a scientific and fancy term for metabolism. The more you exercise the higher your energy expenditure is and the higher your metabolism is!

In addition to doing cardio work we encourage our patients to do some resistance training. Following bariatric surgery, patients lose a significant amount of fat but also lose lean body mass. In order to gain the "good" weight back or to build your lean body mass you need to exercise on a regular basis and perform what we refer to as resistance training, using light weights. The recommendation is to do resistance training 2 or 3 times a week in addition to your cardio workout.

Now if you ask me what type of exercise a patient should be doing I will say that we do not really know which type of exercises work best for our bariatric patients and it truly doesn't matter. What matters is that bariatric patients should exercise!

I encourage bariatric patients to do anything that they like and enjoy, such as jogging, weightlifting, cycling, swimming, or even walking. What is important is for you to get out there and enjoy your life and be active. You have worked hard to get the weight off so now go outside enjoy your life and keep that weight off.

13. AM I GOING TO BE ABLE TO EAT WHATEVER I WANT AFTER SURGERY OR AM I GOING TO BE ON A DIET FOR THE REST OF MY LIFE?

One very common question that I get from my patients is the following: "Dr., after I have my procedure am I going to have to be on a special diet for the rest of my life?"

There is a common misconception that following bariatric surgery patients have to be on a special diet for the rest of their lives. As a matter of fact most patients following bariatric surgery end up eating whatever they want just a few months following surgery with few exceptions and even fewer limitations. Early on after undergoing bariatric surgery, however, patients have to be on a special diet. Most centers have a structured progressive diet which usually starts with liquids and progresses to a blenderized diet and then to a soft diet for a few weeks, after which the patient is allowed to have a regular diet. The notion that the patient will be on a special diet for the rest of his or her life is just a myth!

One must keep in mind that because of anatomical changes following a procedure like a bypass or sleeve or even a band, certain food items may not be well tolerated. These include items like beef, chicken, or even pork. Patients who like to eat those food items usually end up grinding the beef or chicken to make it softer and easier to digest. From talking to my patients over the years I have realized nonetheless that every patient is different and that many patients may be able to tolerate similar food items without any problem.

Early on after a procedure, patients may not be able to eat more than a quarter of a cup or half a cup of food at a time because of all the swelling and inflammation which can lead to a reduced opening. However, with time, patients usually progress to eating 1 cup at a time or even more.

Keep in mind that if you are able to eat anything you want without feeling sick you should not feel that you have a free pass to eat whatever you want and that you are invincible because you had a bariatric procedure and therefore you will not gain weight. That is not true. As I said previously, long-term success after surgery depends on how compliant you are and whether you are exercising or not. When you sign up for bariatric surgery in a comprehensive bariatric center you will meet with the dietician and social worker on multiple occasions prior to undergoing surgery and you will be required to start learning how to make healthier food choices like reading labels, measuring portions, counting calories, avoiding carbohydrates, introducing more protein in your diet, for example, alongside the many other changes to your lifestyle. After surgery you should continue to use these new lessons to be successful in the long run because if you do not you could easily put weight back on. If your surgeon tells you that you can do anything you want because you will never put weight back on then that person is not being honest with you. You must be committed and put some effort into this process otherwise I promise you that you will put some weight back on! (I hate to say it but it's true.) Another thing to keep in mind is that self-monitoring, whether it's by using an app, a food diary or a food journal, is the best way to maintain weight loss following surgery.

Studies have shown that patients who continue to practice self-monitoring by using diaries or apps or whatever other means they have at their disposal, and those who continue to weigh themselves on a regular basis following surgery, tend to maintain their weight loss much better compared to other patients. If you are few months out after your procedure and you are not able to tolerate half a cup or a whole cup of food at once, or if you experience nausea and vomiting every time you have a meal, please inform your doctor to make sure you do not have a stenosis or narrowing of your pouch or outlet.

14. WHY IS BARIATRIC SURGERY CALLED METABOLIC SURGERY AND HOW DOES SURGERY HELP ME WITH MY MEDICAL CONDITIONS?

Bariatric surgery, or weight loss surgery, has gone through many changes over the past few decades. As physicians we did not truly understand why people lose weight after bariatric surgery until recently. In the past we used to think that surgery caused either restriction, whereby it works by limiting the amount of food you can eat; or malabsorption, whereby the absorption of the food you do eat is limited. Based on that very limited understanding we used to divide procedures according to what we thought was the mechanism of action. For example, procedures like a gastric sleeve or gastric band were classified as restrictive, whereas a procedure like a gastric bypass was considered a malabsorptive procedure—because of the malabsorption caused by the re-routing of the bowel as we described in a previous chapter.

With time we came to understand that weight loss after bariatric surgery is not caused by the restriction or the malabsorption alone but by the hormonal and metabolic changes. Many studies have actually shown that following bariatric surgery the main factors leading to weight loss are the hormonal changes that control the appetite and the way the brain processes information and digestion. In simple terms, there is some kind of complex communication system between the gastrointestinal tract and the brain that is mediated through hormones and other factors that control your metabolism and, in turn, weight loss.

Following bariatric surgery, the changes that happen to that communication system change your "set point "and affect your metabolism and energy expenditure to induce weight loss. In addition to the weight loss and because of those hormonal changes in the communication system patients experience an initial very impressive improvement of their medical conditions. That improvement or even cure happens early on in many cases and is not related to the weight loss. If this sounds complicated, I will give you a simple example. When we perform a gastric bypass on a patient who has diabetes type II, the improvement in diabetes happens in the first few days following surgery even before the patient starts losing weight— so that improvement is not dependent on weight loss because the patient could not lose that much weight in only the first few days. To explain this further, following a gastric bypass many gastrointestinal hormones produced by the cells lining your gut like GLP-1, PYY, CCK, Oxyntomodulin, etc. are rapidly released after each meal which, in turn, has profound effects on the brain centers that control appetite and food intake (there is more on this in the weight loss and weight gain centers chapter). This causes rapid improvement in diabetes and also appetite suppression, reduction of food intake and weight loss.

15. WHY CAN'T I LOSE WEIGHT BY JUST GOING ON A DIET?

The answer to this question is very complicated, however the simple truth is that diets do not work. From talking to my patients I have realized that all of the patients I have treated and operated on over the years have been on one type of diet or another and that despite their best efforts they were not able to maintain their weight loss. Everybody loses weight after starting a new diet but maintaining that weight loss is very difficult if not impossible!

I used to keep track of the different diets available and their advantages and disadvantages in order to be able to educate my patients better, such the Atkins diet, South Beach diet, high fat diet, etc. however I stopped doing that because diets do not work and it is a waste of my time and my patients' time. In addition, diets can be very expensive.

We are not talking about patients who need to lose a few pounds; if that is the case then diet and exercise alone are more than enough but if your BMI is higher than 30 or 35 then diets alone will not work. Do not take my word for it, just ask yourself how many times you lost weight on a special diet only to gain it all back shortly afterward. This is called the "yo-yo effect." Researchers have looked into this and realized, after years of animal and human studies, that there is something in our DNA called the "set point." Your body tries to maintain your weight around a certain "set point" by changing your "energy expenditure" which is a scientific term for your metabolism.

If you try to lose weight by, for example, limiting the amount of calories you are consuming on a daily basis through just starving yourself or going on a diet your body energy expenditure goes down in order to prevent you from losing too much weight. So, what ends up happening is that you lose some weight initially and then you stop losing weight and bounce quickly back to your "set point." When you go on a diet and limit how many calories you are consuming your body goes into starvation mode to preserve energy and takes you back to your starting point. If you consume too many calories your energy expenditure goes up and you start burning more so even then it is hard to gain weight beyond your set point. Yes, it is a battle, and unfortunately your metabolism always comes out on top. Now, do not get me wrong! I am not suggesting that consuming fewer calories and exercising is not going to help people who are looking to lose a few pounds because that is quite feasible, I am just saying that people who need to lose 30, 50, 100 pounds or even more, to get down to a healthy weight, will have a much harder time to achieve their goals only because for those patients the issue of weight loss is not as simple as "calories in" and "calories out."

16. HOW LONG DO I NEED TO TAKE MY VITAMINS FOR?

The simple answer to the question of how long you need to take your vitamins for is: for good!

Because of the restriction in the amount of food that patients can eat after surgery and the lack of absorption of all the nutrients and vitamins into the bloodstream, patients are at risk of developing vitamin deficiencies. Therefore, it is very important to be compliant with taking vitamins on a daily basis starting the day you are discharged from the hospital. In the first month or so swallowing large vitamin tablets may cause nausea, dry heaving, or even vomiting because of the inflammation and swelling in your pouch immediately after surgery. It may be very beneficial early on to start with chewable vitamins or even liquid vitamins. After that you can safely start swallowing regular vitamin tablets. However, if you decide to continue with chewable vitamins that is okay too. As a patient you have a choice between taking generic multivitamins or taking commercially available vitamins specifically made for bariatric patients.

Examples of commercially available vitamins:

Bariatric Fusion: This comes as a complete vitamin and mineral supplement, dosed at 4 regular or chewable multivitamins per day. Flavors that are available include orange cream, mixed berry, strawberry, tropical, and wild cherry. If you are anemic or a menstruating young patient you have to add an extra iron pill. Visit www.bariatricfusion.com for more information.

Celebrate: Also comes as a complete vitamin and mineral supplement in either chewable tablets or capsules. Patients taking capsules need 3 capsules per day. Celebrate capsules do not contain calcium or iron so you will need to also take 1200-1500 mg of calcium citrate per day and also daily iron supplements. Patients taking chewable vitamins need to take two tablets per day. The chewable tablets contain iron so no need for extra iron but do not contain calcium so you will need to take 1200-1500 mg of calcium. Visit www.celebratevitamins.com for more information.

Bariatric Advantage: This is a complete vitamin and mineral supplement that comes in capsule form (3 capsules/day) or as chewable tablets in two flavors orange and berry (2 chewables/day.) Bariatric advantage does not contain calcium so you will need to also take 1200-1500 mg of calcium citrate per day. Visit www.bariatricadvantage.com for more information.

Regular multivitamins over-the-counter are also a good option (One multivitamin/day for band patients and 2 multivitamins/day for all other bariatric patients), however regular multivitamins have to be supplemented by 1200-1500 mg of calcium citrate and also daily vitamin B-12 350-500 µg a day.

Patients suffering from anemia or menstruating women who are at risk for anemia should take additional iron above what is provided in the multivitamin. Goal is to take a total of 50-100 mg of elemental iron daily. So please check the iron content of your vitamin brand and supplement as necessary.

There are a few important points to keep in mind.

Multivitamins containing iron should not be taken with calcium. Take at least 2 hours apart to avoid absorption issues.

Avoid children's vitamins because they're usually incomplete. Make sure the multivitamin contains at least 400 µg of folic acid and 18-27 mg of iron.

Patient who undergo biliopancreatic diversion should also take fat-soluble vitamins including vitamin A (10,000IU/day) vitamin D (2000IU/day) and vitamin K (300 µg/day.)

17. IS SURGERY COVERED BY INSURANCE?

One of the most important questions that our patients have when they come to the office for their initial consultation or during information seminars, is whether bariatric surgery is covered by insurance. The issue of insurance coverage is a very complicated one and depends on your specific insurance plan and state regulations. In this chapter I will try to simplify the issue and provide some helpful tips to be able to obtain coverage.

In brief, most insurance companies do cover bariatric surgery as long as the patient has the benefit and meet the following criteria:

BMI of 40, or higher

BMI of 35, or higher with at least one obesity associated medical condition like high blood pressure, sleep apnea or diabetes. Band is approved for patients with BMI of 30 or higher with at least one obesity associated medical condition.

Patients are encouraged to check with their employers, human resource departments or even call the insurance company to make sure that bariatric surgery is covered under their specific plans. Medicare does not require patients to be enrolled in physician-supervised medical weight loss programs prior to surgery but unfortunately some private insurance providers do (usually 3 to 12 months, more on that in the chapter on insurance mandated weight loss programs.)

First, Medicare patients.

Patients who are 65 or older or are disabled are covered by Medicare. In the past Medicare did not cover bariatric surgery, however, over time and after many studies having showed that bariatric surgery is safe in the elderly population, Medicare's policy changed, and bariatric surgery is currently a covered benefit. When Medicare decided initially to cover bariatric surgery, the surgery had to be done in a center of excellence as designated by the American Society of Metabolic and Bariatric Surgery (ASMBS) or the American College of Surgeons (ACS). Because of concerns about access to care, that requirement recently changed, and Medicare patients can now have surgery anywhere they want. However, as discussed previously I would still recommend having surgery in an accredited center whether you are a Medicare patient or not just because we know based on many studies that patients who have procedures in accredited centers fare much better than others!

Sleeve gastrectomy was initially excluded because it was considered an experimental procedure, but sleeve is now covered just like the other procedures. Revisional procedures whether it's for weight gain or because of complications are also usually covered.

Second, private insurance.

Patients who have private insurance have to keep few things in mind:

Not all insurance policies do cover bariatric surgery and even if your insurance company covers bariatric surgery you may not be able to take full benefit of it.

Obesity may be considered a pre-existing condition, check your insurance company policy on pre-existing conditions.

Some insurance companies require the patient to be enrolled in a 3- or 6-month physician-supervised medical weight loss program and multiple consecutive weigh-ins. Some even require a 12-month medical weight loss program to be complete prior to surgery.

You may also have to pay a deductible depending on your insurance policy. In addition, even if bariatric surgery is covered by your insurance you may still have a co-pay.

Every insurance company has a different policy in terms of what is considered an obesity associated medical condition and what is not. For example, high cholesterol may be considered as an obesity associated medical condition by some insurance companies but not others.

One issue that some of my patients encountered and is worth mentioning is that even though their insurance company cover bariatric surgery, their employers chose to exclude bariatric surgery as a covered benefit which means the patients were not covered. In cases like that you have few options:

- Check with your employer or the HR office to see if coverage for bariatric surgery can be added to your insurance plan.

- Switch your insurance to a different insurance provider that covers bariatric surgery.

- Call your insurance to see if you have the option of adding the benefit of undergoing bariatric surgery to your plan.

- Pay out of pocket—not a very good option because a procedure like a sleeve can cost up to $17,000.

Third, health care exchange plans.

If you are covered by a health care exchange plan under the Affordable Care Act (ACA), or "ObamaCare," then you may or may not be covered to undergo bariatric surgery depending on the state you live in. The coverage issue for bariatric surgery in the ACA was left to the state to decide. For example, bariatric surgery is a covered benefit under ObamaCare in New Jersey and New York but is not a covered benefit in the state of Pennsylvania. Currently, only 22 states offer bariatric surgery coverage under its health care exchanges and only 5 states offer coverage for medical weight loss treatment.

The one good thing about the ACA is that dietary counseling and obesity screening is now covered which should raise awareness against the epidemic of obesity in the US.

18. WHAT SHOULD I DO IF MY SURGERY IS DENIED BY MY INSURANCE COMPANY?

This is a very important issue that cannot be covered in its entirety in a single chapter because insurance issues are very complicated, and each insurance company has its own set of policies and guidelines. I will try to concentrate on a few important issues and scenarios and give you some suggestions on what to do if you get denied. Remember that in order to build a strong case and get covered you will need the involvement of all team members in your surgeon's office. The dietitian, social worker, coordinator in addition to the surgeon have to document and submit documentation to the insurance company to demonstrate that you qualify for bariatric surgery. Documents may include copies of your office visits, dietary counseling, psychological counseling, medical or cardiac clearance letter, letter of support from your family physician, copies of your blood work, history of diet attempts, history of weight loss, copies of all endoscopic procedures that you might have had, copy of your sleep study, etc.

It is important to call your insurance company ahead of time to check to see if you have the benefit. Most insurance companies cover bariatric surgery if the patient qualifies based on the BMI and medical conditions (as discussed above) as long as the patient has the benefit. This means your insurance policy should not specifically exclude bariatric surgery as a covered benefit. If that is the case and bariatric surgery is not a covered benefit under your insurance policy it would be extremely difficult to get your procedure covered even if you or your surgeon makes a thousand phone calls to the insurance company. Your best bet in a situation like that is to change your insurance company or talk to your employer to see if the benefit can be added to your policy. This may not happen immediately but when it is time to renew your policy or sign up for new benefits at the end of the year this is something that you can probably get done with minimal or no cost to you.

Now let's discuss some real-life situations and talk about how we can overturn the denial and get you covered. For the sake of this discussion let's say Dr. E. is planning on performing a gastric bypass on a patient named Heather.

Heather gets denied because of incomplete documentation. Believe it or not this happens quite often and is very easy to remedy by asking the surgeon or the team involved to document and send all the necessary documents to the insurance company again. Also, it may not be a bad idea if you call the insurance company yourself and ask what document is missing specifically. In our office we have insurance specialists who do that kind of job, but it won't hurt if you call as well—you are your own best advocate!

Heather gets denied because of incomplete diet history. Again, this can be corrected by obtaining all the documents that show your diet history over the previous few years. These documents can usually be obtained from your family physician office, surgeon's office or any other diet centers that you might have gone to.

Heather gets denied because she does not meet the BMI criteria. If your BMI is less than 35 then you won't qualify (unless you are having a band, the criteria for a band were recently changed to 30 or more.) However, if your BMI was more than 35 when you went to see the surgeon initially for a bariatric procedure and then ended up losing some weight (and now your BMI is less than 35) then you should not be penalized just because you were compliant and were following the instructions of the dietician to eat healthier and ended up losing weight. Your surgeon or somebody in the office should make a phone call and argue that you should not be penalized for losing weight and that your BMI was actually 35 when you first came in. As long as this is documented it should not be a problem!

Heather gets denied because of incomplete documentation of her medical issues. As previously discussed, one of the criteria to qualify for bariatric surgery if your BMI is less than 40 is to have at least one medical condition like high blood pressure or diabetes. If you have diabetes or high blood pressure but that is not clearly documented and there is no mention of the medications, you are taking the case will get denied. In that situation the best approach is to obtain all the necessary documents from your primary care physician who is treating your condition and send it to the insurance company.

Heather was denied because she was deemed non-compliant. Many insurance companies use that excuse in order to make the point that the patient is not trying hard to lose the weight on her own so that means she will not do well after surgery and therefore she is denied. This is an old trick and a lame excuse (to say the least!) This is something that you need your surgeon's office to deal with. Again, it comes down to documentation, so if your surgeon has clear documentation that you were attending the dietary classes and meeting with the dietician and social worker on a regular basis then you can counter that argument and get the denial overturned. If you have actually lost some weight along the process you can also use that as proof that you are actually very compliant and following the instructions of your surgeon and support staff as shown by your 5 or 10 pounds weight loss!

These are just few examples of what we have to deal with on a daily basis. The main thing is not to give up and continue to fight for your right to be treated. You can also ask your surgeon to schedule what we call "peer to peer" with the medical director of your insurance company. This is a last-ditch effort but it works! A "peer to peer" is basically a scheduled phone conversation between your surgeon and the person who decided not to approve your surgery (usually a physician who works for the insurance company.) During that phone conversation your surgeon will basically act like your lawyer and argue your case by explaining to the other doctor why you are a good candidate and why you should undergo surgery by describing your medical condition and how you would benefit from surgery.

19. WHAT DO I DO WITH THE EXCESS SKIN AFTER SURGERY?

This is a very common question that I get all the time—especially from young patients—so I want to emphasize that you should not undergo surgery just to look good (even though I promise you that you will) but to be healthy.

The issue of excess skin after surgery is a very complicated issue because you may or may not have excess skin depending on your initial BMI, age, amount of weight loss, skin nature, how many times you have lost weight over the years, and whether you exercise or not. Either way, excess skin can be easily removed if you decide to do that after you lose the weight. Some bariatric surgeons perform excess skin removal themselves but complicated procedures like removal of excess skin from your upper arms or thighs should be done by plastic surgeons who have more experience in doing those kinds of procedures.

However, keep in mind that removal of excess skin after bariatric surgery is not generally covered by insurance so you will have to pay out of pocket (and unfortunately this can cost thousands of dollars!) Now if you can show that your excess skin is causing some medical issues like skin rashes, skin infections, back pain, neck pain, or skin breakdown then you will have a higher chance of getting the surgery covered by insurance because it will be considered medically necessary. What you will need to work on in this case is documentation, documentation,

documentation! I cannot emphasize that enough. The bigger the paper trail, the better your chance of getting your surgery covered. This should include doctor's notes (from your family physician, plastic surgeon, or even bariatric surgeon) explaining why your doctors think that your plastic surgery is medically necessary. This should be accompanied by pictures and also copies of your prescriptions if possible. So, if you develop a rash or infection don't take any antibiotic or use any medication until you have the rash examined by a physician and documented.

Now the other thing to keep in mind is that removal of excess skin does not guarantee perfect results and a nice six pack (unfortunately it is just not going to happen!) The only thing plastic surgery is doing is exchanging the excess skin for a scar! The surgeon will try to hide the scar, but you will definitely have a scar and it will be a long scar!

One more thing I want to emphasize is that you should not consider plastic surgery until you stop losing weight and you are close to your goal or you have lost most of your excess weight loss—called your plateau. Do wait until you reach your plateau before seeking a consultation with a plastic surgeon (more on the expected weight loss after surgery in the weight loss chapter.)

Some patients are not interested in skin surgery and are not bothered by excess skin so if you are one of those patients then you are good and you don't even have to worry about another surgery especially that skin does not have any negative health implications. Only a small percentage of my patients do undergo plastic surgery and my nurse always tells patients skin won't kill you, but diabetes will!

20. HOW WILL PEOPLE REACT TO MY NEW LOOK AFTER SURGERY?

The simple answer to this question is that people reaction to your surgery will be different depending on the kind of relationship you have with those people. My experience is that people who are close to my patients and truly care about their well-being and health are usually very supportive. However, more distant people who may have a superficial relationship with you or who do not truly care about your health may exhibit a negative reaction toward you especially if they have a weight problem too (but don't ever let it get to your head!) People who care about you (whether your significant other, a friend, or a family member) will make an effort to educate themselves about the benefits of surgery and will encourage you and support you throughout your journey.

Others may not understand the benefits of surgery or the reasons behind your decision to undergo surgery and may therefore react negatively when they see you lose weight. I have a patient who told me that after she lost 100 pounds and felt great she saw a "friend" who told her that she looked sick which made her cry for days. When people react negatively toward you, in my simple opinion, you have two options.

You can just ignore the comments and avoid those people altogether because you do not want to be around negative people who have negative energy. However, if you care about those people and they are truly close to you then you have to make an effort to educate them about the benefits of surgery and about the reasons why you decided to have surgery— explain to them the health benefits of surgery and how important this is to you. My experience is that people who care about you will understand and will come around and support you but, if they don't, then you have your answer and you know what to do!

Another issue worth mentioning is the reaction of people in your community who may have a weight problem themselves (friends or even complete strangers.) Some of those people may be intrigued when they start seeing you losing weight and they may approach you asking to be educated on the process. So, don't be shy, speak up and share your experience. (You can also tell them to refer to Dr. E,'s book for more information if you don't like talking!) However, some people may tell you that you took the easy way out and that you should be ashamed of yourself because while they're working hard to lose weight you got an "easy pass." My experience with those people is that they are either ignorant or simply jealous! So again, if you find it in your heart to spend time with them and explain to them that bariatric surgery is not the easy way out and that surgery does require courage and commitment and hard work to be successful than that is great because you will be doing them a favor. However, if you do not feel like making the effort or the other person is being abrasive and resistant and not willing to listen then I would just avoid them altogether and avoid the negative energy. (Dr. E. is all about positive energy!)

I had a patient whose friend was always giving her a hard time about her decision to have surgery but over time and after she saw how well she did and how healthy she became and after attending some of our support groups she decided to have surgery herself! I can tell you many stories like that but I think you have got my point!

21. WHAT KIND OF SUPPORT DO I NEED AFTER SURGERY?

I always tell my patients that short term success is guaranteed, this means that patients lose weight early on with minimal effort (that's what we call the honeymoon phase!) However, long term success depends on how compliant and how active the patient is. If you are reading this book, then this is a really a great start because that means you are trying to educate yourself so I believe you will be very successful in the long run!

Now, what kind of support will you need? You will need the emotional and social support of your significant other, family and friends, and also the support of your surgeon and his or her supporting staff.

To start, it's very important for you to surround yourself with positive people who care about you and your health. These should be people who understand why you had surgery and support your decision. Sometimes people around you may have a negative reaction to you after surgery, refer to the chapter on relationships to know how to deal with these people!

In addition to that support you will need the continuous support of your surgeon and the team that you met before surgery (coordinator, dietitian and social worker).

Despite the excellent safety profile of bariatric surgery and even though the complication rates following surgery are very low—it's very unlikely for bariatric patients to develop any surgical complications when the surgery is performed by an experienced surgeon in an accredited center—unfortunately bad things can happen, whether it's an ulcer, hernia, or stricture (narrowing of the stoma) and your surgeon should be always available to help you get past these issues.

Also, bariatric patients need the support of dietitians early on and after surgery to review their dietary restrictions and emphasize the need to take vitamins and answer any questions they might have. It is not uncommon for us to ask patients to bring their vitamin bottles with them to the office so that we have our dietitians go over it to make sure our patients are taking the required supplements.

We routinely hold classes and courses for patients who already had surgery to review their dietary requirements and educate them on how to eat healthy, read labels, count calories, and much more—again we are not putting patients on special diets after surgery but we are trying to educate them on healthy eating habits! Your surgeon may not have the time or the expertise to review your food journals but dietitians routinely do that and that's really very important for patients who are trying to maintain their weight loss and for patients who gained weight over time.

If you are not getting that support from your surgeon's office, then you should seek the support from other programs in the area. Sometimes programs have open support groups that welcome patients from outside programs.

The support of social workers is also very important. Some of the patients who undergo surgery have psychiatric issues like bipolar disorder, depression, or anxiety, so the availability of a social worker or a psychologist in a bariatric practice is crucial to provide the much-needed support and follow up. Patients can also develop relationship problems, transfer addiction and struggle with drinking issues or even drugs, so the support of a trained professional after surgery in similar cases is very important to rescue those patients and put them back on track. I always tell my patients that doing surgery is one thing but following patients long term to make sure they continue to do well and get the support they need is a completely different thing, so you need to make sure your surgeon is willing to do the necessary follow ups and provide all the support you need, that is what I do and that's what every bariatric surgeon should do!

22. HOW DO I KNOW IF I AM SUCCESSFUL FOLLOWING SURGERY?

Success after surgery is defined differently depending on the doctor you talk to. In general, success is defined as 50% excess weight loss or more. Therefore, any patient who loses 50% of his or her excess weight or more is considered successful (for a better understanding of excess weight loss refer to the chapter on weight loss.) Patients who lose less than 50% of their excess weight one year after surgery are considered unsuccessful. Even if you don't lose the weight after surgery, do not get frustrated there is still hope and help is definitely available, please read the chapter on failure to lose weight after surgery if you are concerned that you haven't lost enough weight.

Defining success based on weight loss is a very simple way of looking at things but in real life things are way more complicated. I will try to simplify it and give you an insight on how you should truly define success.

Success truly depends on the way we define it. One can argue that improvement in lifestyle and resolution (cure) of the medical issues that are related to obesity following surgery is what defines success (and I have to agree with that!) When I see a new patient in my office the first question I ask him or her is "what are you looking to get out of surgery" because I need to develop an understanding of what the patient is looking for and based on that I can help the patient choose the right procedure and also set the goals and expectations.

For example, if I have an obese patient who is referred to me to undergo surgery because of his poorly controlled diabetes then our goal is to cure his diabetes and not only to make him lose weight. So weight loss is truly a secondary issue and not our main focus. Following surgery, the success of that patient, let's call him David, is based on whether his diabetes is still poorly controlled, is better controlled, or has completed resolved. So, in my opinion, the amount of weight loss in David's case is not essential and should not be used to define success. Are you going to call David a failure if his diabetes is cured but he only lost 40% and not 50% of his excess weight? Of course not, that would be crazy! On the other hand, if David loses 60% of his excess weight but his diabetes—the reason why he came to see me in the first place—is still poorly controlled or completely out of control, then David will feel that he is a failure and that Dr. E. is also a failure—and we don't want that!

I also have many patients who are not interested in weight loss, but they are interested in being physically more active to spend quality time with their kids or grandkids. They want to be able to go shopping without using a scooter or walk in the park and enjoy the summer days. They want to be able to fly without using a seatbelt extender or take rides in amusement parks. They want to be able to bend to tie their shoes or even cross their legs—these things may not mean much to normal patients but for obese patients these are very important aspects of everyday life. If those patients lose enough weight to be able to do just that than they have succeeded and achieved their goals whether the weight loss is 90%, 60% or even 20%.

23. HOW MUCH WEIGHT AM I GOING TO LOSE AFTER SURGERY?

The amount of weight the patient loses after surgery depends on many factors. Your surgeon will not be able to tell you exactly how much weight you will lose after surgery—and honestly it doesn't truly matter that much!—but he or she can give you an idea about the average weight loss depending on two things:

Surgical procedure: For example, on average band or sleeve patients lose less weight compared to bypass patients.

Starting BMI: The higher the BMI the higher the number of pounds you will lose after surgery. However, in terms of percentage, the percentage of weight loss for patients with higher BMI is usually less than patients with lower BMI. I know this is confusing but it's very important to understand that point so I will explain it in a little bit with an example, keep reading!

The way doctors report weight loss is variable. In the past we used to report weight loss based on what we called percentage excess weight loss or % EWL. For example, if I say that the patient excess weight loss is 50% that means that the patient lost 50% of whatever excess weight he or she has. 60% excess weight loss means that the patient lost 60% of whatever excess weight he or she has (makes sense?) Surgeons like to use percentage excess weight loss or % EWL because we can tell patients what the expected percentage excess weight loss is following a specific procedure at each time interval.

For example, Dr. E. performed a gastric bypass on Mrs. Smith who is 100 pounds over her ideal body weight. Mrs. Smith is expected to achieve on average 50% excess weight loss at 3 months. This means Mrs. Smith will lose 50% of her 100 lbs or 50 lbs three months after surgery—not bad, Mrs. Smith!

So, Dr. E., how do you know the ideal body weight of your patient?

The ideal body weights are based on what we call Metlife tables which are tables of average ideal weights for males and females based on the body frame. Not an "ideal" way to determine your ideal body weight!

Another way is to base your calculation on a BMI of 25 (which is a normal BMI). Now this is getting too complicated so I'm going to stop here. But the point I was trying to make is that this is all an approximation so do not expect your surgeon to tell you exactly how much weight you will lose!

Another way of reporting weight loss is by using total number of pounds lost (this does not need any further explanation) or even percentage of total weight loss. For example, a patient weighing 200 pounds who achieve a 5% total weight loss means they lost 10 pounds.

We can also report weight loss based on your BMI loss (or even percentage BMI loss), for example if you start with a BMI of 50 and go down to a BMI of 30 your BMI loss is 20.

Now let's go back to % EWL (percentage excess weight loss) and tell you how much Dr. E. expects you to lose following each procedure.

To start, the procedures that result in the lowest amount of weight loss are gastric banding and gastric balloon.

The procedures that result in the highest amount of weight loss are sleeve gastrectomy, gastric bypass, and duodenal switch

(less than 1% of the procedures done in the US are duodenal switch so we will not concentrate on that procedure here.)

On average, excess weight loss with the gastric band at 12 months is around 30% to 50% at most in the best hands. However, I'm not a big fan of the band because weight loss is inconsistent, and some patients lose no weight whatsoever. Even patients who are happy with their weight loss do develop long-term complications which we talked about previously.

The excess weight loss with a gastric balloon is around 25% at 6 months but to keep the weight loss after the balloon is removed at 6 months you are expected to continue to follow the dietary restrictions, lifestyle changes, and also be active.

The excess weight loss following a gastric bypass is on average 50% at 3 months, 60% at 6 months and 70% at 12 months.

A simple way to remember that is 50, 60, 70 at 3, 6, and 12 months.

The weight loss following a sleeve gastrectomy which is the most commonly performed procedure now in the US as we previously said is on average 15-25% less compared to a gastric bypass (but still much better than the band or balloon!) So the weight loss is on average 40% at 3 months, 50% at 6 months and 60% at 12 months. So again, a simple way to remember that is 40, 50, 60 at 3, 6 and 12 months.

For example:

- Dr. E. performs a sleeve gastrectomy on Mrs. Smith, and Mrs. Smith is 100 pounds overweight.

- Mrs. Smith's expected weight loss is 40 lbs at 3 months, 50 lbs at 6 months, and 60 lbs at 12 months. (Dr. E. reminds you that Mrs. Smith will continue to lose weight up to 18 months and if she is very active and compliant, she will definitely lose more than the average.)

- If Mrs. Smith decides to have a gastric bypass instead then her expected weight loss is now 50 lbs at 3 months, 60 lbs at 6 months, and 70 lbs at 12 months.

Keep in mind two things:

1. The decision to have a sleeve or a gastric bypass or any other procedure should not only depend on the expected amount of weight loss after the procedure because other factors like age, BMI, and associated medical conditions should be taken into account.

2. The lower the BMI the smaller the difference in weight loss between sleeve and bypass, so a patient with a BMI of 36 for example is expected to lose the same amount of weight whether he or she undergoes a sleeve or bypass at least in the short-term (long term weight loss and success is a different issue and is addressed separately in a different chapter!)

24. WHAT IS DUMPING?

Dumping is something that patients ask about all the time but rarely experience. Back in the old days dumping used to be more common but nowadays its becoming less frequent just because we are doing a better job I think as doctors educating our patients about dumping and how to avoid it especially since we have a better understanding of what causes it.

From talking to my patients, I know that dumping is not truly a big issue and patients learn how to avoid it quickly.

So, what is it?

Dumping is your body's reaction to simple sugars or sweets like chocolate or dessert—what we call simple carbohydrates. When people experience dumping they develop rapid heartbeat (the heart starts racing), they become sweaty, dizzy, and light-headed. Patients tell me that it feels like they are having a heart attack. Some people even have the runs! There are two types of dumping depending on the timing.

Early dumping happens within the first 30 minutes after eating and this is usually because of the gush of fluids from inside your vascular system into your gastrointestinal tract or gut which causes the drop in blood pressure hence the dizziness, lightheadedness, etc.

Late dumping happens hours after eating and this is more complicated in physiology, but I will try to make it simple here. What usually happens in late dumping is that your blood sugar goes up quickly because your blood is absorbing the sugar that you ate so your body overreacts by secreting a big load of insulin which in turn causes your blood sugar to drop. The drop in blood sugar can cause some of those symptoms we mentioned earlier with the heart racing and feeling sweaty, etc., just like when a diabetic experience a drop in blood sugar. If you are a diabetic, then you know exactly what I am talking about.

There is a rare metabolic form of low blood sugar that happens more than one year after a gastric bypass that is called medically "postprandial hyperinsulinemic hypoglycemia." This disorder is very similar to late dumping and causes the same symptoms. So, if you develop those symptoms we talked about please tell your doctor. This is usually managed with some dietary changes and in extreme cases medications.

Dumping is usually seen in gastric bypass patients but is less frequent following a sleeve or duodenal switch because in those cases the "pylorus" or the exit gate of the stomach is preserved!

One thing I need to emphasize is that your decision whether to have a bypass or not should not be based solely on the risk of dumping because like I said it's not common and you can learn how to avoid it quickly. Also, gastric bypass is still the "gold standard" and can result in excellent long-term weight loss and cure of many medical conditions especially diabetes! So, if you are a patient who has a high BMI and suffers from diabetes for example you should strongly consider having a gastric bypass without being discouraged by dumping. I have patients who are completely against having a gastric bypass and when I ask why is that, they say, "Oh, gastric bypass causes dumping, I don't want it!" Believe it or not, some patients do like the fact that they experience dumping because they feel like dumping keeps them honest and makes them avoid food items that they should not be eating in the first place—sugars and sweets.

25. WHY DO I HAVE HEARTBURN AFTER MY SLEEVE?

Even though sleeve gastrectomy is a very safe and effective procedure, long-term issues like heartburn and weight gain do happen. We talked about weight gain in a different chapter so I will concentrate on heartburn here. Heartburn is the sensation of burning in the chest or all the way up in the throat which can happen months or even years after surgery. This is what doctors call Gastro Esophageal Reflux Disease or GERD just in case you hear that term! Doctors do not know exactly why sleeve patients develop heartburn after surgery but we have few explanations. Keep in mind that in some cases heartburn goes away after a sleeve gastrectomy especially with weight loss but that is not always the case.

So why do people have heartburn after a sleeve? Dr. E. will answer—or at least try to!

First, after performing a sleeve gastrectomy and because of anatomical changes, the sphincter of the lower esophagus, which is the entrance site to the stomach, stays open for longer periods of time which can result in gastric juice going up in the opposite direction to the esophagus or even the throat—and believe me gastric juice burns, hence the heartburn!

Another explanation is that the pressure inside the gastric sleeve is so high it pushes the gastric juice up into your esophagus all the way up in the chest. Remember that when surgeons do a sleeve gastrectomy they cut out 80% of your stomach so you are left with a much smaller stomach but with a much higher pressure, so you go from a high volume, low pressure system to a low volume, high pressure system, yes—it's just like plumbing! One thing worth mentioning is that some people do not describe heartburn but regurgitation, which means they bring undigested food up mostly when they are lying flat at night! Even though this is different than heartburn and harder to treat (as we will discuss in the next chapter) it's due to the same problems that we see after a sleeve gastrectomy which cause heartburn, specifically the opening of the sphincter and the high pressure inside the gastric sleeve.

If you have heartburn before undergoing a sleeve gastrectomy you may or may not develop heartburn afterward! I know this is becoming confusing but please bear with me! Let's say you have a hiatal hernia which is a large opening between your chest and abdomen through which your esophagus enters your abdomen and connects to the stomach. The hiatal hernia itself can cause heartburn and even pain, especially when large in size. So, if your surgeon fixes that hernia when doing the sleeve you probably won't have any heartburn afterwards or it will be less likely. However, if you have heartburn without an anatomical problem to explain why you are having heartburn in the first place then having a sleeve may cause the heartburn to get worse (you can still have the sleeve but that's a risk you are taking).

If I see a patient whose heartburn or GERD is truly bothersome or if the patient has severe inflammation of the esophagus because of heartburn then I usually recommend a bypass instead of a sleeve. Also, if you have a condition called Barrett's esophagus—a pre- cancerous condition caused by severe inflammation in the lower esophagus—then most surgeons would not do the sleeve but a gastric bypass instead. if you have Barrett's esophagus and your surgeon tells you that you can have the sleeve then you must run the other way!

26. WHAT DO I DO IF I HAVE HEARTBURN AFTER BARIATRIC SURGERY?

The incidence of heartburn after bariatric surgery depends on which procedure you had. For example, following a gastric bypass it is very unlikely for patients to complain of heartburn, however following a sleeve gastrectomy or duodenal switch, people can develop heartburn even years after surgery. We did talk in a previous chapter about why patients develop heartburn after a sleeve so I'm not going to discuss that again, but I will concentrate on what to do when the patient comes back with heartburn.

After a gastric bypass just like I mentioned previously heartburn is uncommon so when the patient comes to the office complaining of heartburn or regurgitation I usually recommend an upper endoscopy or an EGD to make sure that the patient does not have inflammation of the gastric pouch, ulcer, or even stricture (narrowing of the opening of the pouch.) If the endoscopy does not show any problem the patient is usually given a prescription for a proton pump inhibitor (PPI)(e.g. Nexium, Prilosec, Protonix, etc.) or anti-acid drug. In most patients PPI is usually enough to manage the heartburn. Sometimes sucralfate (Carafate) is also prescribed. If that doesn't work then the issue becomes more complicated and your surgeon will have to look for anatomical reasons behind your heartburn and regurgitation (like a problem with the way the bypass was performed in the first place but this is beyond the scope of this book.)

After a sleeve gastrectomy heartburn is more common and usually the first line of treatment is again PPI plus or minus sucralfate (Carafate.) Doctors usually start with a low dose once daily but can go up to twice daily if you are still not getting any relief. In addition to medication you will be required to make some changes to you eating habits and your daily routine, so make sure you talk to the dietitian and follow the recommendations. For example, instead of eating 3 meals per day you will be required to eat multiple smaller meals to give your gastric sleeve the chance to empty and avoid regurgitation. You should also try not to eat and go to bed or lay flat immediately afterward. I usually ask my sleeve patients who have heartburn to wait for at least an hour after having a meal before lying down to avoid any heartburn. In addition, your surgeon may order a special test to document the presence of heartburn especially if they are not sure if it's truly heartburn or something different (a 24-hour catheter-based study or a wireless probe study called Bravo®) but because heartburn is common after a sleeve I have to admit that most surgeons start the medication empirically (i.e. without ordering any fancy tests to make the diagnosis.)

In extreme cases of heartburn or regurgitation especially when the medications are not working patients may have to undergo a sleeve conversion to a different weight loss procedure like a gastric bypass (i.e. the surgeon will take down the sleeve and perform a gastric bypass instead.) If you haven't lost enough weight with a sleeve and you are having severe heartburn then a conversion to a gastric bypass may sound like a good idea because it will take care of the heartburn issue and also result in more weight loss!!! On the flip side, however, we have many patients who are very satisfied with the weight loss after a sleeve but not happy about the heartburn issue and for those patients we usually offer a non-invasive endoscopic procedure called Stretta® to strengthen the sphincter of the esophagus which as we previously discussed is responsible for the heartburn or a surgical magnetic sphincter augmentation procedure called LINX. Either way, make sure you talk to your doctor and discuss all the available options, the medical and the surgical ones!

27. DO I NEED TO TAKE ANY MEDICATIONS AFTER BARIATRIC SURGERY?

The simple answer is no!

The purpose of undergoing bariatric surgery is to lose weight and be healthy and stop taking medications altogether!

You will need to take vitamins, however, this is very important and was discussed in a separate chapter.

Keep in mind that in certain cases your surgeon may ask you to take certain medications if you develop inflammation of the gastric pouch, inflammation of the esophagus, heartburn (just like we discussed in the chapter on heartburn), or if you develop a complication like an ulcer after a gastric bypass. However, even then you will have to take the medication only for a specific period of time and when your condition resolves the medication can be discontinued.

Now to avoid any problems following surgery especially after a bypass or duodenal switch many surgeons (including Dr. E.) will start a Proton Pump Inhibitor (PPI) prophylactically for a few months (prophylactically means that the medication is given to avoid any problem down the line and not because we are treating a specific condition.)

Studies have shown that if you give PPIs to patients after a gastric bypass for a few months (up to 6 months) then the chance of patients developing an ulcer goes down significantly!

Examples of PPIs are: Prilosec, Nexium, Protonix, Dexilant, Zegerid, Kapidex, etc

Keep in mind that you do not want to take those drugs forever because they have their own side effects like osteoporosis, pneumonia, or even colitis (inflammation of the colon.) If you are doing well after bariatric surgery and are not having any issues you don't need to take any of those medications after the first few months!

Many of these medications are over the counter so you can buy them without a prescription, however always ask for a prescription and check with your insurance company to see if it's covered by your insurance. It is wise to try to save some money on these medications in order to spend it on your vitamins which are rarely covered by insurance!

28. HOW SAFE IS SURGERY AND WHAT ARE THE POTENTIAL COMPLICATIONS?

The quick and easy answer is: very safe!

One thing I always tell patients is that bariatric surgery is now, because of all the technological advances and special training, as safe as gallbladder surgery—if not safer.

When surgeons started doing bariatric surgery on a large scale in the '80s and '90s, the surgery was done in an open fashion (by making a large incision in the abdomen to access the inside of your body) and the complication rates were high. People were developing surgical site infections, hernias, and other complications and were also spending up to a week in the hospital because of pain and slow recovery.

With the advances in technology we started doing the procedures laparoscopically (using keyhole surgery) by making small incisions and using long instruments and a camera to access the inside and this truly revolutionized the way we do things. At the same time, the procedures became standardized and surgeons started establishing what we call centers of excellence, or accredited centers, where doctors and other health care providers are especially trained to take care of bariatric patients.

We also started collecting data to see how we are doing as doctors and also find ways to improve the outcome of our patients. All of this led to bariatric surgery becoming one of the safest surgeries out there!

One thing to keep in mind before signing up for surgery is that you need to do some research when you choose your surgeon and your program (as we mentioned in the previous chapters) because the chance of you developing a complication is usually lower in experienced hands and in accredited centers. I truly believe that if you choose a good surgeon and go to a reputable center you will do very well and the chance of developing a complication will be really very low.

So how low is low?

In general, the chance of developing any complication following bariatric surgery in accredited centers is less than 5%. Some places do better than others so please check your program website for information on outcomes and complications or even ask your surgeon. Also, the chance of developing serious complications like hemorrhage or staple line breakdown (leak) is even lower than that and is usually around 1–2%.

Some complications are non-specific, which means they can happen with any kind of surgery and these are:

- surgical site infection: i.e. wound infection for which you may have to get antibiotics or even get the wound opened and drained and sometimes even packed to keep it clean. This is obviously less common with laparoscopic surgery because the incisions are much smaller to start.

- DVT: Deep Vein Thrombosis means blood clots in the legs. It can happen with any kind of surgery but patients undergoing bariatric surgery are at higher risk compared to other patients so you will most likely receive an anti-coagulation drug before surgery (like heparin, lovenox, arixtra, etc.) and most likely afterward as well to prevent DVT. If you are at a very high risk of developing DVT (because of a coagulation disorder for example) or if you had a DVT in the past you doctor may decide to give you anti-coagulation for a prolonged period of time after surgery (like one week or two)or even place what we call a filter or screen to prevent the development of an embolus or pulmonary embolus (PE).

- pneumonia: infection of the lungs

- pulmonary embolus: clot traveling from the legs to the heart and lungs, can be life threatening but is also preventable with anti-coagulation and early walking

- dehydration: secondary to poor fluid intake

- nausea and vomiting: can be the result of anesthesia or the over usage of pain medications after surgery, can be prevented by limiting the use of narcotics and also the use of anti-emetics (meaning anti-nausea medications)

- bleeding: can happen with any kind of surgery but more so with bariatric surgery, talk to your surgeon about your specific bleeding risk and please mention if you can receive blood transfusions or not if need be. If you are a Jehovah's Witness make sure you tell your surgeon, some bariatric surgeons will not operate on Jehovah's Witness patients.

- cardiac events: like irregular heartbeat or even heart attack because of the stress of surgery, your surgeon will make sure you undergo medical and cardiac testing and clearance before surgery to prevent any cardiac complication.

Other complications are specific for bariatric patients:

- leak: meaning gastric juice leaking out of the confinement of the gastric pouch or the lumen (inside) of your gastrointestinal (GI) tract. This is a dangerous and life-threatening complication but fortunately leak is uncommon. The treatment of a leak requires a prolonged hospital stay, antibiotics, the use of intravenous nutrition, or even another operation.

- obstruction: this happens when you develop a blockage in your GI tract because of a technical issue at the time of your procedure or because of bleeding and the formation of a blood clot that acts like a plug. Sometimes an obstruction develops over time because of a narrowing in your GI tract. This complication, again, is uncommon but usually results in nausea and vomiting, abdominal pain and the inability to eat, drink or keep anything down. It's more common with a bypass but it can also happen with a sleeve (where it's usually called stenosis of the sleeve) or even a band if your band is too tight.

- fistula: a fistula is an abnormal connection between two organs. One of the common fistulas that we encounter in bariatric surgery is a fistula between your pouch and your old stomach (called remnant) following a bypass. A fistula in that case can cause pain, inflammation of the pouch, ulcer and yes, weight gain. Depending on your symptoms a fistula can be managed with medications or another operation to take it down.

- ulceration: usually happens to gastric bypass patients. it can occur because of NSAID medications (like aspirin, ibuprofen, etc.), H.Pylori infection, a very large pouch that is producing too much acid, or even a fistula but above all it happens in smokers! (So please, please, please do not smoke!) Ulcers are usually treated with anti-acid medications like proton pump inhibitors (PPI) and also sucralfate (Carafate.) In special circumstances patients may have to undergo surgery if the ulcer is not healing with medications.

- vitamin deficiencies: vitamin deficiencies are uncommon if you are taking your vitamins but can happen once you stop taking your vitamins. Vitamin deficiencies can cause many symptoms like fatigue, weakness, numbness, tingling, or even anemia. If you start developing numbness and tingling please call your doctor immediately because this can be a sign of vitamin B1 deficiency and the damage to the nerves can become permanent very quickly.

- anemia: this can happen because of poor iron absorption especially after a bypass, mini-bypass, or duodenal switch. Therefore, iron supplements after surgery is very important. Young menstruating women are a high-risk group of patients and may require an extra dose of iron and even intravenous iron infusions sometimes.

- dumping: please refer to the chapter on dumping.

- hair loss: is usually transient, happens during the initial rapid weight loss phase after surgery (honeymoon phase) and can be prevented by taking protein supplements and also biotin.

29. IS WEIGHT LOSS GOING TO HELP MY SEX LIFE?

This is a question that I don't get often because many patients are shy and therefore embarrassed of bringing the issue up. I decided to include it in this book because I believe that it is a very important issue.

Obesity results in poor quality of life and sexual dysfunction in both males and females, but mostly in females which in turn can affect their relationships with their significant others.

It is well known that obesity is associated with many medical conditions like diabetes, elevated blood sugar, elevated cholesterol level, and joint pain. In addition to these medical issues, and to make matters even worse, studies have shown that obesity results in poor quality of life and sexual dysfunction in both males and females. Elderly females are at particularly high risk because of low estrogen levels.

It is estimated that more than 50% of obese women suffer from some form of sexual dysfunction, like pain during or after intercourse, in addition to loss of sexual desire or drive. Obesity can result not only in your inability to have sex because of your medical issues but also in the loss of your sexual desire and drive altogether. Sexual dysfunction in women is not only present in obese females but also in females suffering from other medical conditions, however, obesity makes this problem much worse.

Many studies have also shown that sexual dysfunction or no sex at all in obese females results in social problems and affects the quality of lives and relationships.

Following bariatric surgery, the weight loss achieved may result not only in a significant improvement in your medical conditions but also in your sex life.

Many studies have looked into this very sensitive issue and found that after surgery patients report better sexual desire and also better sexual performance which in turn improves their relationships. The other interesting thing in these studies is that the improvement in sexual function was independent of the type of surgery or the amount of weight loss. Even a small amount of weight loss or improvement in medical conditions after surgery go a long way in improving patients' sex lives.

So, if you are morbidly obese and suffer from sexual dysfunction you may want to consider the impact that the excess weight has on your health and sexual life and consider having bariatric surgery. I believe that bariatric surgery may improve not only your health and sexual life but also your relationship with your significant other. This is what bariatric surgery is truly all about: not weight loss per se, but a significant improvement in your health and lifestyle.

30. WHAT KIND OF TESTS DO I HAVE TO HAVE BEFORE SURGERY?

Before you undergo bariatric surgery, your surgeon will ask you to undergo some testing. Keep in mind that most patients who undergo a routine procedure have to have some kind of testing such as blood work and echocardiogram. Prior to bariatric surgery you may have to undergo some additional specific tests that may be required by your insurance company or by your surgeon just to make sure you are safe to have surgery.

Here is an example of these tests:

- Blood tests: these tests usually include vitamin levels to check and make sure you don't have any vitamin deficiencies. (Dr. E. recommends repleting any vitamin deficiency prior to surgery.) Vitamin D deficiency is quite common in obese patients so don't feel bad if your surgeon tells you that you need to take a high dose of vitamin D prior to surgery. Blood tests will also include a lipid profile as a baseline and also iron studies to make sure you are not anemic and don't need iron supplements before surgery. On multiple occasions we had to give patients who were found to be severely anemic iron infusions prior to surgery.

- Chest X-ray: this is truly an old practice and even though many doctors don't see a huge benefit in getting

101

a chest X-ray before surgery (including Dr. E.!) many insurance companies, hospitals, and anesthesiologists continue to request it.

- EKG: electrocardiogram to make sure you do not suffer from any arrythmias or heart issues; if there is any abnormality you may be required to undergo additional testing like a nuclear stress test, 2D echocardiogram, or even cardiac catherization

- Sleep study: many centers send their patients for a sleep study to rule out sleep apnea given the high incidence of sleep apnea in the obese patients. A sleep study can be done in specialized centers or at your home.

Some other centers, like ours, perform a screening test based on a questionnaire called STOP BANG (there is a range of questionnaires available) to screen for sleep apnea. Patients who are found to be at high risk are then referred for a sleep study.

- Cardiac/medical clearance: you will be required to obtain a medical clearance to make sure you are fit for surgery from your medical doctor or a cardiologist who will examine you, review your tests, and decide whether you are a good candidate for surgery. In the past we used to use the term "cleared for surgery" but now what medical doctors do is assign a risk category to the patient based on the individual risk factors like age, medical conditions, etc., so patients are usually assigned to one of three categories: low risk for surgery, intermediate risk for surgery, or high risk for surgery. Intermediate or high risk for surgery doesn't mean you can't have surgery; it only means that your chance of developing a complication following surgery is higher than the average patient.

- Upper endoscopy: many surgeons do require that you undergo an upper endoscopy prior to surgery to make sure there are no issues that can cause a problem during surgery like tumors, polyps, ulcers, etc. Keep in mind that surgery is performed on the upper part of your gastrointestinal tract and during surgery your surgeon doesn't necessarily look inside the lumen of your stomach or small bowel so it makes sense for your surgeon to look inside prior to cutting or stapling your stomach. During the endoscopy a biopsy is usually taken to rule out Helicobacter Pylori (a bacteria that lives in the stomach and can cause severe inflammation or even ulceration.) Some centers will ask for an upper gastrointestinal series (X-ray of your stomach and small bowel taken after you are asked to drink a contrast material) instead of doing an upper endoscopy. If you are older than 50 and never had a colonoscopy you may also be required to undergo a colonoscopy ahead of time.

- Helicobacter Pylori testing: usually involves a blood test or a stool sample. If you are undergoing an upper endoscopy, then a biopsy will be most likely taken at the same time to rule this out.

- Arterial blood gas (ABG): this is not a standard test, but it may be required if you have any pulmonary issues.

- Pulmonary function tests: this is not a standard test unless you suffer from a pulmonary condition like Chronic Obstructive Pulmonary Disorder (COPD) or emphysema. It may also be required by insurance companies in certain cases.

If you are having surgery, you may be required to have some or all of the above tests but do not get frustrated. Tests are important to help your surgeon plan for any potential complication and perform the procedure safely. I always tell my patients: safety comes first!

31. WHY IS MY APPETITE BACK NOW AND WHAT CAN I DO TO CONTROL IT?

Appetite suppression or lack of appetite is something that happens immediately after surgery. There are many explanations for why patients have no appetite after surgery. The first and most common explanation is the drop in the level of an orexigenic hormone, and appetite stimulant called "ghrelin," which is produced by the stomach and controls the appetite center in your brain. We mentioned the communication system between the stomach and brain and this hormone is one way these systems communicate. Appetite suppression happens mostly after sleeve gastrectomy but also after a gastric bypass or a duodenal switch. In addition to that hormonal factor, after surgery patients end up with a much smaller stomach pouch which causes restriction and in turn appetite suppression. In addition to the small size of the stomach itself, after surgery the severe inflammation and swelling that happens in the first few weeks after surgery contribute to the appetite suppression post-operatively. The third factor is the stress of surgery itself. All these factors combined lead to the early period of appetite suppression!

I have to tell you that patients truly enjoy that early phase—hence the name honeymoon phase—because they are not eating much but are still very satisfied and do not feel hungry. In certain cases we have to remind patients to eat their meals! Yes, appetite suppression can do that much!

The challenge for the patients is how to control the appetite after the honeymoon phase. After the first few months (sometimes weeks for some patients) the level of ghrelin goes up again and swelling and inflammation is gone, so the restriction is much less, and the patient is past the stress of surgery. Put all of these together and the appetite comes back!

Now keep in mind, even though the appetite is back the balance is still tipped in your favor—if you remember from our previous chapter, surgery has already changed your "set point" so now your metabolism is working in your favor—but you need to learn how to control the appetite to maximize your weight loss and be successful.

When your appetite comes back do not be discouraged as this is an indication that you are healing well and it is part of the natural process after surgery. The most important thing is not to start grazing to satisfy your appetite because grazing is one of the leading causes of weight gain and it honestly defeats the purpose of having surgery in the first place.

Here is a list of a few things you can do to control your appetite (I learned many of these from my patients, although they are not really scientifically proven they do work!)

Try to drink water in between meals, sometimes hunger is just what we call "head hunger" meaning your brain is asking you to fill your pouch with something and water may just do it for you.

In addition to your three meals add one healthy snack that is rich in protein, for example peanut butter, mixed nuts, dry fruits, etc.

Start incorporating protein bars and protein shakes in your daily routine in between meals.

Go for a walk or run outside.

Sugar-free chewing gum (don't swallow it!)

Occupy yourself with something fun like reading a book, talking to a friend, or even playing video games!

These are just some suggestions, but the main point is that you need to control your appetite one way or another or it will control your life!

32. MY SIGNIFICANT OTHER DOES NOT SUPPORT MY DECISION TO HAVE SURGERY, WHAT SHOULD I DO?

How nice would it be if your significant other supported every decision you make! Unfortunately, this is not always the case. (My wife would tell you that she doesn't always support my decisions!)

I have had the honor of taking care of hundreds of patients who showed up in the office for their initial consultation with a significant other who was very supportive and many times had more questions than the patient himself or herself. Honestly this makes things much easier for the patient and surgeon too because as we mentioned previously you will need all the support you can get after surgery. So if your significant other is on board that is great! Now what if he or she is not?

The main thing to find out is why your significant other does not support your decision. My experience is that it is most probably for one of the following reasons:

1. Your significant other is concerned about your safety. Your significant other knows that surgery will help you lose the weight and get healthy but he or she is concerned about your safety. The fix for this is very easy. Ask your significant other to do some research to find out how safe the procedure is or go with you to meet your surgeon to find out more. If he or she is not will-

ing to do that ask your surgeon to try to reach out (I've made so many phone calls over the years to concerned family members to the point that I developed the habit of asking my patients whether they would like me to reach out to any family member.) If all else fails buy them a copy of my book!

2. Your significant other does not truly understand the seriousness of obesity. In that case you need to make an effort to educate your significant other about the benefits of surgery and why this is so important to you and your health. Again, if you can convince him or her to accompany you to the surgeon's office or to a support group to listen to some stories and talk to other patients that would help a lot.

3. Your significant other has a weight issue too but cannot find the courage to have the surgery or support you in your decision. Your best bet in this case is to try to convince your significant other to have the surgery if they qualify by explaining how this can help you both and also help your relationship. I have operated on many couples in the past (sometimes on the same day) and I found out that couples often do better than other patients because they support each other and keep each other honest. Following surgery, couples who undergo surgery together (from what they tell me) experience a significant improvement in their relationship, their interactions with others, and their sex lives. Even their kids start eating healthier and become more active.

4. Your significant other may be concerned that the change in your external look may have a negative effect on your relationship. I have many female patients tell me that

their husbands are against them having surgery because they are concerned if they lose weight and look better they may leave them! If that's the case I recommend an open conversation about your relationship before undergoing surgery. I have seen many couples break up after surgery because of issues of this kind. If you have marital problems then unfortunately surgery will not help, in fact, it might make it worse (I hate to say it but it's true and I have seen it in the past).

In such a case you should probably seek marriage counseling before surgery.

If you look hard enough you will find that your significant other's reasons for not supporting your decision to have surgery fall in to one of those four categories. Please try to have an open conversation and listen to each other carefully to find out what the issue is and see if you can convince him or her otherwise.

33. HOW SOON CAN I GO BACK TO WORK?

The downtime after surgery is usually 2 weeks as long as the operation is done laparoscopically. If you have an open procedure—an open procedure is when your surgeon makes a large incision in your abdomen to obtain access to your stomach and bowel—the downtime may be longer. Keep in mind that the downtime varies depending on your age, medical conditions, the type of procedure you are having, and how well you recover after surgery.

As previously mentioned, patients who undergo laparoscopic surgery recover faster than other patients. Band patients are usually treated as outpatients—meaning they leave the hospital the same day after surgery—whereas patients who undergo other procedures, like sleeve or bypass, end up staying for 1 to 3 days in the hospital as their recovery usually takes longer. Also, younger healthier patients recover faster than older patients who suffer from medical conditions like high blood pressure, diabetes, sleep apnea, etc.

If you have a desk job or work from home and you want to go back to work sooner, you should talk to your doctor to check and see if you can do that. I usually let patients go back to work before the end of the 2-week period as long as they are off of their pain medications, are able to tolerate their liquid diet, and are taking their vitamins. The issue is that vitamins, the special diet (liquid diet), and pain medication can be overwhelming in the first week or so after surgery so before you are given a release to go back to work your surgeon wants to make sure you are doing well and following the instructions.

Also, in the first few weeks after surgery patients are usually very sleepy and tired and even though I encourage patients to be active early on they may need to nap during the day so we do not want you to go back to work early while you are still feeling run down!

Driving is another issue, we usually tell patients not to drive until after their first postoperative office visit to make sure they are recovering well. It also goes without saying that you can't drive while taking your pain medication! Always check with your surgeon before driving again!

In the unfortunate event that you develop a complication after surgery—which as mentioned above is very uncommon— you may need to spend a few more days in the hospital and be off work for longer than 2 weeks, and until your surgeon feels that you are safe to go back to work. Patients who need to take more than a few weeks off from work may need to submit short-term disability paperwork to their employer when necessary, and your surgeon's office should be able to help you out with that. I am hoping you won't have to, though!

34. HOW BAD IS MY PAIN GOING TO BE AFTER SURGERY?

Overall, the pain after surgery is not bad, especially if you undergo a laparoscopic procedure where incisions are usually very small. Patients who undergo an open procedure end up with a bigger incision and usually have more pain that must be managed with intravenous pain medications for a few days at the hospital.

Different patients have different pain thresholds, so some patients take minimal to no pain medications and others have to get a refill of their pain pills.

Pain medications that are usually prescribed include: Percocet, Vicodin, Tylenol #3, etc.

Pain after bariatric surgery when performed laparoscopically is two-fold: in the first few hours after surgery patients usually describe diffuse abdominal pain, bloating, and even shoulder pain. This is usually due to the gas used to develop a space inside your abdomen in order to perform the surgery. In addition to taking pain medications the one thing that can truly help is walking! Surgeons usually encourage patients to walk immediately after surgery to help with gas pain and also prevent the development of blood clots in the legs.

The other kind of pain is incisional pain around the small incisions used to perform the surgery. This kind of pain is sharp and localized to the incisions and this is usually managed with pain medications. Keep in mind that with robotic surgery incisions are usually smaller and cause less pain. Also many surgeons are now performing blocks during bariatric procedures to avoid postoperative pain.

Pain medications used in the hospital are mostly narcotics (like morphine or dilaudid). These medications are effective but can cause side effects including nausea and vomiting, so if your pain is not too bad ask for non-narcotic pain medications like plain Tylenol. Other non-narcotic pain medications that are available are intravenous Toradol (ketorolac), which is an NSAID that can cause bleeding or even affect your kidney function so some surgeons (including Dr. E.) prefer not to use it, especially early on after surgery. Another medication that is effective and recently became available is intravenous acetaminophen (Ofirmev), which is the intravenous form of Tylenol. This is a safe and effective medication but is expensive and not available in all hospitals.

One thing worth mentioning is that after you are discharged from the hospital your pain should get better with time so if your pain is not getting better, or is getting worse, this may be an indication that there is something wrong and you need to call your surgeon immediately.

35. WHAT SHOULD I EXPECT DURING MY HOSPITAL STAY?

Hospitals have different protocols and ways of doing things. However, many accredited bariatric centers follow more or less similar pathways in managing patients before and after surgery. Some variations may occur.

The day of your surgery you will be admitted and evaluated by an anesthesiologist who you may or may not have met in your preparation for surgery. Your surgeon will also greet you before you are taken to the operating room. You will most likely receive intravenous antibiotics and a subcutaneous injection of a blood thinner like heparin or other commercial products (like Lovenox or Arixtra) to prevent deep vein thrombosis (blood clots) in your legs during the operation. After the operation you will be taken to a dedicated floor and will meet the nursing staff that will take care of you during your hospital stay.

Depending on your surgeon's preference you may or may not wake up with a surgical drain in your abdomen and a Foley catheter in your bladder. Nasogastric tubes (NGT) are rarely used nowadays in bariatric patients. The surgical drain is usually left in place for safety reasons in case you develop a breakdown of the staple line in order to control any leakage or infection.

Most surgeons have stopped using these drains, especially since bariatric procedures are becoming one of the safest abdominal operations (talk to your surgeon ahead of time and ask if a drain will be used or not). I do not routinely use any drains unless the procedure is a revision. Foley catheters are usually left in place to monitor your urine output, but they are placed while under anesthesia and they should not cause any discomfort once you are awake. Foley catheters are usually removed on postoperative day 1.

After surgery you will be asked to walk on a regular basis like we mentioned previously to prevent any blood clots in the legs and you will be also asked to use an incentive spirometer (a blue breathing device that you suck air through) to prevent atelectasis (collapse of your lungs) and to help avoid pulmonary complications and fevers.

After surgery you will be started on a clear liquid diet of water, broth, and jelly a few hours after surgery, or the day following surgery depending on your surgeon's specific protocol. In some centers, including ours, patients are started on a liquid diet 6 to 8 hours after surgery without performing any radiographic studies or X-rays. In other centers surgeons order an Upper Gastrointestinal Series (UGI) which is basically an X-ray taken after you are asked to drink some contrast to make sure there is no leakage of contrast outside your pouch before starting you on the liquid diet.

You will also undergo blood work on the day of surgery and the day after to check for bleeding and make sure you don't have any electrolyte disturbances or kidney problems. If you suffer from chronic medical conditions it is very likely that you will be evaluated by your family physician, an internist or a hospitalist to manage your medical conditions during your hospital stay.

During your hospital stay you will also be monitored very closely for any potential complications and if there is any suspicion that you may have developed a problem based on a rapid heart rate (called tachycardia) abnormal blood work, or abnormal physical exam you may undergo further imaging studies or even a diagnostic or therapeutic re-exploration.

Diagnostic re-exploration means your surgeon may decide to take you back to the operating room to make sure you don't have a problem whereas a therapeutic one is usually to correct a problem or manage a complication of surgery.

Blood transfusions are very uncommon but may be required if you develop bleeding or hemorrhage. If you are a Jehovah's Witness or if your religious beliefs prevent you from accepting a blood transfusion you must let your surgeon know ahead of time.

If your hospital stay goes smoothly you will be discharged within 1 to 3 days depending on your specific condition and the specific operation you have had. Prior to discharge, your Foley will be removed but your drain (if you have one) may or may not be removed, however. Some patients are discharged with surgical drains, which will later be removed in the office. The bariatric coordinator or the dietitian will review your diet and the nursing staff will review your discharge instructions. Prior to discharge the medical team will also review your medications and make the appropriate adjustments. The patient's medications are usually switched from long-acting to short-acting because of malabsorption and patients are asked to cut or crush the tablets for at least one month after surgery. After that any pill up to the size of an M&M can be taken whole.

36. WHAT SHOULD I BE EATING IMMEDIATELY AFTER SURGERY?

The postoperative diet or the diet that you will be on for few weeks after surgery is usually what we call a progressive diet. The dietitian of your bariatric program and your surgeon should review that diet with you before the operation and also on the day of discharge.

A progressive diet stands for a diet that progresses over time from liquids to other food items with different textures, usually over three or four stages.

You will find that different centers have different diet progression guidelines but the main principle remains the same: start with liquids, slowly progress to a pureed or blenderized diet (baby food) and then to a soft diet before you go back on a regular diet.

Keep in mind that what I am describing here is just an example and that the time frames are just suggestions, some people can be advanced faster than others whereas others have to be on a liquid diet for longer. Also, your surgeon may put you on a different diet or give you a different diet schedule depending on your specific condition. For example, patients who develop an ulcer or a narrowing of their stoma may be maintained on a liquid diet for much longer to prevent pain, nausea, or vomiting.

Keep in mind few things:

- The most important thing in a postoperative diet is to stay hydrated. One of the main issues we have with bariatric patients is dehydration and we need to avoid that! You may not be able to gulp or chug water after surgery so you have to continuously sip water every 30 minutes or so to stay hydrated, especially early on after surgery when your pouch is swollen and inflamed and you cannot tolerate more than one or two ounces at a time.

- You need to drink around 48 to 64 ounces per day (1.5–2 liters.) This does not have to be water alone—all fluids count. Believe it or not, some patients do not like the taste of water immediately after surgery!

- It is recommended that you supplement your diet throughout these stages with protein shakes, they can provide you with the much-needed protein and fluid content which would count toward your 48–64 ounces.

At our center we use the following diet for all patients who undergo bariatric surgery:

Stage 1: Liquid diet

This is the first stage and usually patients are placed on Stage 1 diet for a week. Liquid diet includes but is not limited to the following:

- G2® sport drinks (low carbohydrates and sugars)
- Crystal-lite®

- water, vitamin waters (different flavors but again watch for the sugars)
- broth
- Jell-O (sugar-free)
- unsweetened iced tea, decaf tea, skim milk (good source of protein as well)

You may need to experiment with different flavors and options to find something that fits you well and does not make you nauseated or sick to your stomach. Always check with your dietitian for ideas and more options if need be.

If you are doing well with the liquid diet, don't get too excited and jump to Stage 2 before the end of the week because you may get sick! Stick with the schedule!

Stage 2: Pureed diet

A pureed diet is anything that is blended and has the consistency of baby food, pudding, or apple sauce. It goes without saying that you can blenderize anything. You will be on Stage 2 for another week. Please keep in mind that if you are having trouble with Stage 1 and are unable to keep the liquid down or get enough liquids in one day you should probably talk to your doctor or dietitian before moving to Stage 2.

Here are a few important things to keep in mind:

Start eating three meals per day (start with ¼ cup.) Develop the habit of measuring your food if possible. You will start with ¼ cup but eventually move to ½ cup and then 1 cup three times daily after the first few months.

- Try not to drink and eat at the same time, this will help you concentrate on getting enough protein during your meals and prevent weight gain in the future. Drinking in between meals or taking protein supplements as a snack when your appetite is back is encouraged!

- Eat very slowly. Take your time and enjoy it!

- You may dislike certain flavors and develop new appreciation for other flavors. That's ok, your taste buds are changing and will continue to change—so go with the flow! I have many patients, for example, who have told me that they used to love chicken and now they can't stand the smell of it!

- Examples of a pureed diet include: apple sauce, cottage cheese, hummus, scrambled eggs, blenderized meat such as chicken or even pork, oatmeal, and pudding, etc.

Stage 3: Soft diet

This is usually the last stage before you go on a regular diet and should last for at least 6 weeks or even longer if you are still having problems with texture and still experimenting with different food items. I think learning how to eat and what to eat is the hardest thing that patients face after surgery, so be patient, take your time, continue trying new things, and above all ask for the help and support of your surgeon, dietitian, or even friends who have had the surgery too. Examples of soft food are eggs, fish, ground beef, tuna, very well-cooked vegetables, etc. Again, stick to some rules:

- Chew your food very well. Remember that your stomach used to do that for you (the stomach is like a mill) but now that you have only a small pouch you have to do it yourself.

- Eat three meals per day and supplement them with protein shakes if need be. Do not skip any meals even if you don't have an appetite.

- Continue experimenting. If you don't like ground beef now you may find it very tasty next week—your taste buds will be playing tricks on you!

- If you do not usually like fish, then please try to! Fish is really great in Stage 3 because it's very soft, it does not require that much chewing, and is very rich in protein. Fish should be your new favorite food!

After the successful completion of your third stage, your surgeon will restart you on a regular diet. At this point you will have hopefully developed some healthy eating habits and gotten used to measuring your food. You are also ideally avoiding drinking and eating at the same time. You will be able to eat anything you want in small portions with some restrictions. A few tips to keep in mind in order to be successful in the long-term and avoid weight gain are:

1. Avoid carbohydrates like rice, bread and pasta—you will be able to introduce some good carbohydrates over time like brown rice, whole grain bread, and pasta, but in very small quantities.

2. Continue to avoid eating and drinking at the same time.

3. Concentrate on foods rich in protein (fish, ground beef, etc.)

4. Increase the amount of food you are eating progressively (1/4 cup to ½ cup to 1 full cup three times daily). If you are counting calories, you may be only consuming 800–1200 calories per day but over time, you should be consuming 2000–2500 calories/day. If you are losing too much weight talk to your doctor because you may need to consume even more than 2500 calories per day.

5. Avoid carbonated beverages. Yes, even diet sodas are a no!

6. Drink coffee and tea in moderation to avoid dehydration.

7. Avoid alcohol because it can get you drunk very easily after bariatric surgery.

8. Do not ever smoke!

9. It is okay to add spices to your food but in moderation.

10. Drink plenty of fluids (at least 48-64 ounces/day.)

11. Start introducing healthy snacks in between your meals, such as protein bars or protein supplements, especially when the appetite comes back. Mix your protein with water or skim milk. Avoid making smoothies because they can contain a lot of sugar even when you use fresh or frozen fruits.

37. WHY DO I HAVE TO LOSE WEIGHT BEFORE SURGERY?

Although you can have surgery without losing any weight pre-operatively, most of the reputable, accredited centers and comprehensive weight loss programs—which is where you should be having your surgery performed—will require that you lose a certain amount of weight preoperatively.

We are not talking here about the mandated 3- or 6-months physician-supervised diets that some insurance companies request before approving your surgery. As we discussed in a previous chapter that requirement imposed on us by some insurance companies is truly not necessary or beneficial and is not based on any scientific evidence. In addition, it can cause a high attrition rate, meaning that patients get sick of the process and drop out altogether, which is why I believe insurance companies have created it in the first place. Yes, some insurance companies would rather not pay for your surgery even though it will make you healthier and less likely to get sick in the future!

The weight loss we are talking about here before surgery is the weight loss that is usually requested by your surgeon before undergoing surgery and it's usually 5–10% of your weight depending on your BMI. Different centers have different weight loss criteria and if your BMI is not high and close to 35 you may not be required to lose any weight at all.

The two main reasons why bariatric surgeons ask patients to lose weight are:

1. Your surgeon wants to make sure you are committed to making some lifestyle changes and that you are compliant with the dietary instructions. At our center we ask patients to implement some specific meal plans and to make changes to their eating habits like avoiding carbonated beverages, measuring food, counting calories, reading labels, using small plates, introducing protein supplements, and not drinking while eating. These changes let patients practice good and healthy eating habits before surgery and are really helpful in making the transition to the postoperative diet after surgery. In addition, we need to make sure that patients are compliant and are able to follow and understand the instructions. We also ask patients to start a physical exercise program. We found that patients who start making these small changes early on lose weight quickly, which tells us that they are ready for surgery!

2. The second reason is a technical reason: when you gain weight on the outside you also gain weight on the inside meaning that your liver becomes much larger than the liver of a patient with a lower BMI because of fat deposits inside the liver. When you gain weight, your liver becomes a storage place for all the extra fat cells, which can lead to what we call medically non-alcoholic steatohepatitis (NASH), which can lead to inflammation and cirrhosis. The purpose of preoperative weight loss is for your liver to shrink so that the surgeon can access and operate on your stomach safely. Many studies have shown that when you lose weight the surgery becomes technically easier and safer so weight loss before surgery is truly very important. Safety comes first!

38. WHAT MEDICATIONS SHOULD I AVOID AFTER SURGERY AND WHAT ABOUT MY DAILY MEDICATIONS?

Before we discuss which medications to avoid after surgery it is important to remember that after surgery you should always discuss with your family physician whether you need to continue or not any medication that you are taking for high blood pressure, high cholesterol, diabetes, etc. The goal is to eventually take you off all medications but that may take some time; in the meantime, your dosages may have to be adjusted.

Also, immediately following surgery and for at least 4 to 6 weeks all medications have to be crushed or cut into small pieces using a pill cutter or crusher to avoid impaction in your pouch which may cause a blockage. After that any medication that is equal or smaller than an M&M can easily be swallowed. In terms of what medications, you need to avoid the simple answer is non-steroidal anti-inflammatory drugs (NSAID). NSAIDs can cause inflammation and even ulceration of your pouch following a gastric bypass or duodenal switch (less common after a sleeve gastrectomy or gastric banding). Here is a list of some over the counter NSAIDs and the brand names:

- Aspirin (Bayer, Excedrin)
- Ibuprofen (Advil, Motrin)
- Naproxen (Aleve)

Prescription NSAIDs include:

- Ketorolac (Toradol)
- Mefenamine (Ponstel)
- Celecoxib (Celebrex)
- Diclofenac (Voltaren)

If, after the first few months following surgery, you really need to take an NSAID for few days for severe back pain, joint pain, or any other reason, it may be okay to do so but always talk to your doctor first. It may also be a good idea to take a PPI (Proton Pump Inhibitor) in the meantime to avoid any inflammation or ulceration in your pouch.

Always check with your surgeon or family physician before taking any new medication as absorption is usually affected (except for gastric banding). Your doctor may not have all the necessary information on a specific medication so enlisting a knowledgeable pharmacist who is willing to research a specific drug (pharmacists are very good at looking up specific drugs) is the smart thing to do. One thing to keep in mind is that, in general, capsules or any other long-acting medications are usually not absorbed very well following bariatric surgery and have to be changed to a short acting medication.

Common cold medications over the counter are safe to take and these include:

- Benadryl
- Robitussin
- Sudafed
- Tylenol (including extra-strength)

Constipation is also very common after bariatric surgery and I usually tell my patients that most of constipation medications over the counter are safe for bariatric patients including:

- Colace
- Dulcolax suppositories
- Fiber products
- Fleet enemas
- Gas-x
- Glycerin suppositories

39. CAN I DRINK ALCOHOL AFTER SURGERY? AND WHAT ABOUT SMOKING?

Drinking alcohol after bariatric surgery can cause serious problems and should be avoided! I know you will not like hearing that especially if you enjoy an occasional glass of wine.

The issue with alcohol is that after a gastric bypass alcohol is usually absorbed very quickly and enters into your blood stream without any processing in your stomach. Normally, alcohol is broken down in the stomach, but after bariatric surgery, the stomach is bypassed. Also, normally after the alcohol enters in your blood stream it goes for additional processing in your liver. After a bypass, however, the enzyme that breaks down alcohol is not as active, so the breakdown process is slower. That creates a two-fold processing problem for alcohol. Not only is the alcohol getting into your bloodstream faster it is also not being broken down as fast as it would have been before bariatric surgery. As a result, the effect of alcohol is much more pronounced, and you can get drunk very easily. Driving Under Intoxication (DUI) is a real risk even after a drink or two.

The effect of alcohol after a sleeve or band is not very well known because there have not been any studies to look at that issue specifically but I usually tell my sleeve and band patients what I tell the bypass patients: avoid alcohol at all costs but if you decide to drink make sure that you remember that the effect of alcohol on you will be much more pronounced. Never drink and drive!

Smoking also is a big NO! I am not going to talk about the bad things that smoking can cause like lung cancer and heart disease because I am sure you know that by now. The issue of smoking in bariatric patients is different. We talked in a different chapter about how safe bariatric surgery is and it is true, bariatric surgery is very safe! But if you are a smoker the chance of you developing a complication like an infection, pneumonia, or, even worse, a postoperative ulcer after a bypass is much higher than in non-smokers.

Therefore, I do not personally operate on smokers unless they quit just because I hate to see any patient develop a complication—like I always say, safety comes first! Also, if you are smoker and you are considering bariatric surgery this is a real opportunity for you to quit and turn your life around. Ask your surgeon about a referral to smoking cessation counseling or talk to your family physician about nicotine patches or even Chantix.

40. CAN I GET PREGNANT AFTER SURGERY?

Of course, you can! I have a patient who gave birth to healthy triplets after undergoing IVF and you can imagine how much fun we had when she brought her kids to the office!

Many studies have shown that patients who get pregnant after undergoing bariatric surgery are less likely to develop pregnancy-related complications that can affect the mother and the fetus like gestational diabetes, preeclampsia, premature delivery, need for a C-section, etc.

The reason why the mother does better when she gets pregnant after losing her excess weight is because she is closer to her ideal body weight and has no obesity-associated medical conditions. Being in a state of better health overall will have a positive impact on your pregnancy.

Most centers, including ours, have monitoring and protein and vitamin supplementation protocols in place for the management of bariatric patients who get pregnant. If you are pregnant or planning on getting pregnant talk to your surgeon and your obstetrician about it. In addition to more frequent blood work to check your vitamin levels you may need to undergo frequent prenatal ultrasounds.

However, we usually warn our patients not to get pregnant in the early phases after surgery when they are still losing weight and have not reached their plateau yet—until their weight has stabilized. The issue is that we do not want our patients to be under the stress of pregnancy while they are still losing weight and are trying to adapt to their new lifestyle. Saying that, I have many patients who did get pregnant immediately after having surgery and did fine, however they were considered high risk patients and we had to follow them very closely and monitor their vitamin levels and the growth of their babies on a regular basis. The safest thing to do is to wait until your weight loss stabilizes before getting pregnant.

41. WHAT IS ROBOTIC SURGERY?

Performing surgical procedures using robotics is a new approach that is now very popular with one procedure performed, somewhere in the world, every 30 seconds. Although robotic surgery was initially used in Urology and Gynecology, this new and exciting technology is now also being used in Bariatrics.

As previously mentioned, laparoscopic surgery has truly revolutionized the way we perform bariatric surgery and has resulted in better outcomes and less pain, so patients are doing much better and are much happier compared to the days of open surgery. Robotic surgery is now the next wave and is poised to replace laparoscopic surgery over the next decade or so. Robotic surgery is sometimes referred to as Da Vinci surgery in reference to the Da Vinci robotic platform that is marketed by Intuitive®, the company that has the largest market share in medical robotics. During robotic surgery, the surgeon sits at a console and operates through small incisions using tiny instruments. The robotic system translates every hand movement the surgeon makes into instrument movements.

Robotic surgery is performed through small incisions in the abdominal wall just like laparoscopic surgery, but the incisions are smaller and there is less torque on the skin which can translate into less bruising, better healing and potentially less pain. Also, the instruments used in robotic surgery are completely different than laparoscopic instruments. Robotic instruments have the added advantage of being wristed instruments so they can move in all directions just like the wrist of human beings as compared to the laparoscopic instruments which can only move in two planes. In addition, robotic surgery allows surgeons better visualization.

The difference between laparoscopic and robotic surgery is like the difference between regular movie theaters and 3D movie theaters, meaning surgeons can see better and perform better. In addition to all those advantages, instruments used in robotic surgery are now taking advantage of artificial intelligence by providing real time feedback for surgeons to help them make sound decisions during surgery, this can potentially translate into better outcomes.

Although I am a big fan of robotics for all the reasons I mentioned previously and although I perform robotic surgery on a regular basis, patients need to know that the use of robotic surgery in bariatrics is still new so patients who are interested in robotic surgery need to do some research in order to find bariatric surgeons who are trained on using this new and exciting technology. Also, my patients seem to think every time I mention robotic surgery that the procedure will be performed by a robot and not me which is not the case. The use of robotics is not meant to replace surgeons but to give surgeons complete control of the operation and enhance their capabilities, so although the surgeon may not be standing by the patient's bedside during the operation, the surgeon is still performing the entire operation from the console or the cockpit!

42. HOW CAN I MAINTAIN MY WEIGHT LOSS AFTER SURGERY?

To be perfectly honest, maintaining weight loss is one of the biggest issues we have to deal with following bariatric surgery. I always tell my patients that maintenance of weight loss following surgery is more labor intensive and much harder than losing weight in the first place.

As previously mentioned, following bariatric surgery patients experience a lot of metabolic and hormonal changes that help with resetting the metabolism and the "set point" that we talked about, therefore weight loss initially seems to happen naturally. Somehow your body seems to want to lose weight early on in order to get down to a healthier weight so that's really good and very encouraging!

However, after the first two years patients start to hit a plateau and in some cases, they start gaining weight. Now before we go any further, I want you to understand that not everybody experiences this weight gain so please do not assume that you will automatically gain weight two years after surgery because that's not the case. Also, some weight gain in the range of 5–10% after the first two years following surgery is not unusual, actually it is to be expected and that kind of weight gain should not be distressing or alarming. The issue is when patients continue to gain weight above that 10% mark.

Now to start, the worst thing you can do if you start gaining weight is to get frustrated, discouraged and not talk to your doctor or surgeon about it. Follow-up is very important after any kind of bariatric surgery. If you are routinely following up with your surgeon talk about your concerns and about your weight gain but if you haven't seen your surgeon in some time, then maybe now it's time to get back on track and see your surgeon again.

The issue of weight gain after surgery is very complicated and I can probably write a whole book just on weight gain alone. Briefly, weight gain can be due to anatomical issues with the surgery itself behavioral issues related to eating and lack of exercise or even your hunger and weight gain center in the brain trying to compensate and take over your metabolism to make you put some weight back.

Many studies have looked into the issue of weight gain following surgery and the different ways to help prevent weight gain and maintain weight loss. The consensus is that the best way to maintain weight loss over time is to exercise and to continue to self-monitor your weight and dietary intake. Popular means to monitor dietary intake is using web based platforms or even apps on your smart phone; popular examples are MyFitnessPal, Spark people, Lose it! Calorie King and Weight Watchers.

Weighing yourself is also important to keep yourself honest, you don't have to weigh yourself twice a day or even every day but regular frequent self-weighing—once or twice a week for example—is very important. An important study based on a national registry have shown that successful weight loss maintainers are the ones who monitor their diet regularly, exercise, eat breakfast daily and practice frequent self-weighing. So how often do you need to exercise?

The recommendation is to exercise for 200–300 minutes per week to maintain weight loss; I know this may be too much, but the plan should be to start slow and build up over time. Exercise does not have to be very intense; I actually recommend less vigorous, lower intensity exercises to avoid injury or harm. Also, if your goal is to do 30 minutes in one specific day you can split that into two separate sessions that are 15 minutes each, the effect will be additive and you are more likely to complete both sessions compared to a single more intense session of 30 min!

Resistance training (using weights for example) and protein intake is also very important for building lean body mass and maintaining weight loss because lean body mass can result in more calorie burning.

43. SHOULD I TAKE ANY WEIGHT LOSS MEDICATION AFTER SURGERY?

The simple answer is NO. The purpose of undergoing weight loss surgery is to avoid the need to take weight loss medications and for the most part bariatric patients do extremely well following surgery and do not need to take any weight loss medications. However, as previously mentioned in a separate chapter, exercise and self-monitoring are very important tools for maintenance of weight loss following bariatric surgery.

Despite the high success rate following bariatric surgery a small number of patients fail to lose an adequate amount of weight or start gaining weight over time (referred to in scientific journals as recidivism or more simply weight regain) and because of that a new approach called "adjuvant pharmacotherapy" have become now popular among surgeons and obesity specialists.

Adjuvant pharmacotherapy is basically the use of FDA-approved weight loss medications, or in certain cases off-label use—off-label use means that the medication is not being used for the reason it was developed in the first place—of certain medications to enhance weight loss following bariatric surgery. The use of medications following surgery to enhance weight loss should only be done under the close supervision of your surgeon or obesity specialist. Selection of the appropriate medication and timing of administration are very important aspects of "adjuvant pharmacothera-py." In addition, those medications need to be closely monitored for side effects (more on that in the pharmacotherapy chapter). The use of medications or "adjuvant pharmacotherapy" should be accompanied by an intensive lifestyle intervention, involving again calorie restriction, self-monitoring and exercise, and behavioral counseling to reinforce good eating habits and healthy choices.

44. WHAT ARE THE WEIGHT LOSS MEDICATIONS THAT ARE AVAILABLE TO ME?

Questions about weight loss medications are probably among the most commonly asked questions even though they are not routinely used in bariatric centers because of price, side effects and limited efficacy.

There are a few principles regarding weight loss medications that patients need to keep in mind. First, the FDA has strict guidelines on the use of anti-obesity or weight loss medications and therefore only patients with BMI ≥ 30 or BMI ≥ 27 in the presence of obesity related health conditions (like diabetes, high blood pressure or sleep apnea) should be prescribed anti-obesity medications. Also, to be effective, those medications need to be utilized in conjunction with what we call "comprehensive intensive lifestyle intervention" preferably under the supervision of trained health care professionals like obesity specialists, dietitians and social workers in addition to exercise specialists. The goal being 5-10% of body weight loss within 6 months.

Patients should not get the impression that they can lose 80 or 90 lbs. with anti-obesity medications because that is unreasonable. Also, the use of medications outside of comprehensive weight loss centers and without the supervision of professionals and without a diet and close follow up doesn't usually work!

The other thing that should also be mentioned before we discuss the different weight loss medications is that weight loss medications should never be given to pregnant patients or patients trying to become pregnant. Currently we have 8 FDA approved weight loss medications (previously 9 before lorcarserin was taken off the market)

The 5 FDA-approved weight loss medications that are most commonly used are:

1. Phentermine:

- One of the most commonly prescribed medications, first approved in 1959, low potential for abuse (controlled substance IV)
- Only approved for 12 weeks although many physicians prescribe it for longer
- Side effects include rapid heart rate, high blood pressure, insomnia or inability to fall asleep, tremors and headache
- Common brand names in the US: Lomaira® and Adipex-P®

2. Orlistat:

- Needs a prescription like the other medications but the lower doses (60 mg) are approved to be purchased over the counter without a prescription (ALLI®)
- Works by blocking the fat absorption in the gut

- Side effects include: oily discharge with flatus (can be very bothersome), gallstones and kidney stones. Needs to be taken with multivitamins
- Common brand name: Xenical®

3. Liraglutide:

- Injectable medication that works by suppressing your appetite and delaying stomach emptying, it also improves blood sugar levels (the medication was initially developed to treat diabetes and continues to be used in lower doses as an anti-diabetes medication)
- Required dose for weight loss is 3.0 mg injected in abdomen, thigh or upper arm any time of the day irrespective of mealtime
- To avoid side effects it's prescribed in increasing doses over 5 weeks starting at 0.6 mg up to 3.0mg (comes in pre filled syringes): week 1 (0.6mg), week 2 (1.2mg), week 3 (1.8mg), week 4 (2.4mg) and week 5 (3.0mg)
- Side effects include nausea, diarrhea, constipation, vomiting, headache, low blood sugar or even pancreatitis (inflammation of the pancreas)
- Should not be used in patients with family history of thyroid cancer
- Common brand name: Saxenda®

4. Phentermine/Topiramate

- This drug is a combination of two drugs phentermine and Topiramate, the thinking being that phentermine can help with short-term weight loss and Topiramate can help with long-term weight loss as well as weight loss maintenance.
- Schedule IV drug
- Take once in the morning with or without food
- Start at 3.75mg/23mg and titrate up to 15mg/92mg
- Side effects include birth defects, numbness, kidney stones, glaucoma, confusion, inability to sleep, irregular heart rate, abnormal taste, and dry mouth.
- Common brand name: Qsymia®

5. Naltrexone/Bupropion

- Combination of naltrexone (used to treat addictions) and bupropion (used to treat depression and smoking cessation)
- Side effects include nausea, diarrhea, constipation and headache.
- Should not be used in patients taking pain medications
- Monitor for suicidal thoughts
- Common brand name: Contrave®

Other less commonly used medications for weight loss are Topiramate (Topamax®), Metformin, Burpopion (Wellbutrin®) and Zonisamide; these are not specifically used for obesity but they can be used off-label by physicians for weight loss, especially after bariatric surgery.

Topiramate and Zonisamide are anti-epileptic drugs that can cause weight loss as a side effect. Metformin is a diabetes medication that can help with weight loss in patients taking medications for depression or psychosis. Bupropion is an antidepressant that can also help with weight loss especially in smokers or patients with anxiety or depression.

Please note that Lorcarserin (Belviq®), a previously FDA approved anti-obesity drug, was withdrawn from the market on February 13, 2020 because of the cancer risk so we are not going to discuss it here.

45. WHAT IS THE ENHANCED RECOVERY PROTOCOL IN BARIATRIC SURGERY AND HOW DOES THAT HELP ME?

Enhanced recovery is a new protocol for taking care of bariatric patients that is now being utilized in most of the accredited bariatric centers. This new protocol was based on a national study that was championed by the American Society of Metabolic and Bariatric Surgery (ASMBS) in order to decrease postoperative pain, improve patient outcomes and also decrease readmissions. In brief, patients are required to drink high-protein drinks the night and morning before the operation to avoid dehydration and prevent muscle breakdown, patients will also be given a cocktail of pain medications, by mouth, once at the hospital immediately before the operation to avoid postoperative pain.

During the operation most surgeons will also perform what we refer to as "TAP block" which is basically the use of numbing medications to numb the nerve endings supplying the abdominal wall; again, this is to avoid postoperative pain and help patients walk quickly and go home sooner. Our results with this new protocol have been very good and we are big proponents of this protocol and I encourage you if you are having surgery to discuss it with your surgeon because you will definitely be happier and recover quicker postoperatively if your surgeon uses the enhanced recovery protocol.

46. WHAT IS WEIGHT BIAS AND HOW CAN WE FIGHT IT?

As previously mentioned, patients who suffer from obesity are commonly subjected to derogative and unjust behavior. All of us have watched TV shows and movies or even witnessed real-time instances where patients who suffer from "obesity" were vilified and treated unfairly or even brushed aside and ignored as if they were not human or do not exist. I can count many examples of such behavior, but I am sure you know exactly what I am talking about.

Many people think that "obese" patients are lazy, unproductive, or even stupid, which is very distressing and heartbreaking to say the least. This kind of behavior is due to what we refer to as "weight bias" and it is something that we need to recognize and try to change. Studies have shown that even physicians have some implicit bias against patients with obesity and tend to spend less time counseling them. Everyone needs to understand, including doctors, that obesity is not the result of poor choices or unhealthy life style, obviously unhealthy eating and lack of exercise can contribute to weight gain, but obesity as such is a disease like heart disease, diabetes and cancer.

I always prefer to say, "patients with obesity" instead of saying "obese patients" even though I do, on occasion, catch myself saying "obese patients." We need to make a consciousness effort to fight "weight bias" and treat any patient with obesity with respect, love, attention and care just like any other patient with a chronic illness.

47. WHAT IS THE ROLE OF SOCIAL MEDIA IN FIGHTING OBESITY?

For better or for worse, social media has become a huge part of our daily lives and although I am not personally a big fan of social media, I am very active on multiple social media platforms. The reason I am not a big fan is because I believe social media makes people spend more hours per day looking at their phones or computer screens instead of socializing so in that sense I think social media is anti-social!Now you are going to be asking: "So, Dr. El Chaar, if you think social media is anti-social why are you so active on social media?" The simple answer is that I am using that very powerful tool in order to reach the thousands of patients I have operated on to keep them engaged, committed, and educated on the pandemic of the century—I am not talking about COVID-19 but Obesity. Many surgeons have actually become healthcare influencers (I am not claiming to be one, but I do my best) and are very active on social media. This is something they should be congratulated on because they are using those platforms to educate and help their patients. Many physicians spend countless hours answering questions in live sessions with their followers to discuss health issues and this is truly a great thing; it is like having a town hall meeting with your doctor instead of your politician.

Therefore, I encourage any patient to try to follow his or her surgeon if they are active on social media in order to stay engaged and educated. If your surgeon is not into social media you can always try to find some reliable accounts run by healthcare professionals with good credentials to follow so that you can learn about healthy eating habits and making good choices postoperatively in order to maintain your weight loss.

Many bariatric programs also have their own Facebook pages and forums for patients. Despite some issues that we had in our program in relation to those social media platforms we have been able, like many other bariatric programs, to harness the power of social media with the implementation of some basic rules. We are able to benefit our patients and develop a culture of camaraderie and friendship where patients feel free to share their experiences and learn from each other.

48. WHY ARE OUR KIDS BECOMING OVERWEIGHT?

The issue of obesity in children and adolescents is heartbreaking to say the least. As a parent this is something that is truly very concerning to me and if your child has a weight issue, I am sure you will feel the same.

According to certain estimates, close to 40% of children and adolescents now are either overweight or obese and although the overall obesity rate may have reached a plateau the number of children with severe (class 2 and 3) obesity is rising rapidly. Unfortunately, children of African-American and Hispanic parents are disproportionately affected by this pandemic.

The risk of obesity in children starts at conception. Pregnant mothers with a weight issue or with diabetes are more likely to have children with a weight issue, so there is a clear association between maternal weight and risk of obesity in children. This is why I tell my patients that when you lose weight your children become healthier and have a lower chance of having a weight issue as adults—so by losing weight you are helping the entire family to lose weight. Also, both very low weight and very high weight babies can develop obesity in the future. Nobody truly knows why certain children are affected by obesity while others are not. Obesity experts believe that "epigenetics" play a role. What is "epigenetics?" Epigenetics is when the environment influences gene expression, meaning that certain environmental factors, such as lack of physical activity, toxins, junk food, chemicals, etc., can switch on the "obesity" genes and cause the child to gain weight over time. In addition to that we now know that there are many disease states in children, like endocrine disorders, that can cause weight gain. Common examples are thyroid or adrenal gland disorders.

Many medications (especially antipsychotic drugs, anti-depressants, prednisone and oral contraceptives) can cause weight gain in children. Very early onset of obesity (in children less than 2 years old) should also make you suspicious of an underlying genetic disorder like MC4R mutation (found in 6% of children with severe early onset obesity), POMC deficiency or leptin deficiency. If the child has some abnormal features, we also consider syndromes like Prader Willi, Laurence Moon, Beckwith-Wiedmann and Alstrom … etc. but those are uncommon.

Parents and care givers do not need to remember all of these names but need to learn how to identify the problem and to report it to the pediatrician and obesity specialist. To start, it is always wise to discuss the issue of weight with the pediatrician if you are concerned that your child is gaining too much weight. Parents and physicians should not feel uncomfortable discussing the weight of children because if we deal with it early on and intervene promptly, we can prevent the child from suffering from obesity as an adult.

The way obesity is defined in children is different than adults. Although we use BMI to classify adults, in children we use growth charts (WHO charts when <2 years old and CDC charts for children 2 to 19). Any child whose BMI is higher than the 85th percentile based on those growth charts is considered overweight and any child who BMI is more than 95th percentile is considered obese. We also have three different classes of obesity based on the BMI percentile. This is important for the provider but not as much for the parents

In brief:

> Healthy weight: BMI<85th
> Overweight: BMI>85th percentile
> Obese Class I: BMI ≥95-120th percentile
> Obese Class II: BMI 120-140th percentile
> Obese Class III: BMI >140th percentile

Our job as parents is to shield our kids from the "toxic" environment that we live in, including the impact of media and the aggressive marketing of calorie dense food whether its fast food, sodas, candy, cereals … etc. Believe me, as a parent I know it's not that easy.

The proliferation of fast food restaurants and the fewer healthy options available to us add to the fact that healthy food in general is way more expensive than the widely available less healthy options; these are factors that work against us but we need to try our best to teach our kids how to make healthy choices and avoid junk food.

In addition to that I would also like to give you some helpful tips to combat obesity in children, those are things that you can practice and institute at home. You may not be able to implement all of them at once, however small changes over time can go a long way. These were based on the recommendations of a panel of obesity experts and include:

1. Screen time (whether it's TV, iPhone, iPad or video games) less than 2 hours per day

2. Active play time at least 60 minutes per day

3. Family mealtime (eat together as a family at least 5–6 times a week)

4. Breakfast daily

5. Daily fruits and vegetables (2 cups for 2yo, 4 to 5 cups for > 2yo)

6. Adequate sleep time for at least 8 hours

7. Avoid eating out

8. Avoid sweetened beverages (juices, sodas ... etc.)

49. IS IT TRUE THAT THE APPETITE CENTER IS IN THE BRAIN AND NOT THE STOMACH?

The issue of appetite is a very important issue because it can help us understand how weight is controlled. Historically, many people used to think that patients with "big" stomachs have a big appetite and therefore eat more and gain weight whereas patients with "small" stomachs have small appetites, so they eat less and do not gain weight. That is exactly why, I believe, that every time I operate on a patient the first thing they ask me is: "How big was my stomach?"

"Big" and "small" stomachs are only a myth because as a matter of fact most people have more or less the same size stomach whether they weigh 100 pounds or 600 pounds. Appetite is controlled by an intricate communication system between the gastrointestinal tract or "gut" and the brain, and not by the size of the stomach.

I will explain further: the brain (more specifically, the arcuate nucleus of the hypothalamus) has two centers, one is responsible for weight gain (bad center) and is called ARP/NPY and the other one is responsible for weight loss (good center) and is called alpha-MSH/CART. The ARP/NPY center causes weight gain by increasing food intake and stimulating the appetite whereas the alpha-MSH/CART center causes weight loss by decreasing food intake and suppressing the appetite. Therefore, the effect of stimulating the "bad" center is weight gain whereas the effect of stimulating the "good" center is weight loss!

Now what stimulates those centers? Those centers are stimulated by hormones and factors released by cells lining the gut in response to environmental factors, food, and even surgery, as previously mentioned. Ghrelin for example (which is produced by the stomach) is what we call an "orexigenic" hormone, or appetite stimulant, because it stimulates the "bad" center and causes weight gain, whereas other hormones like GLP-1, PYY, CCK, Leptin … etc. are considered "anorexigenic" because they stimulate the "good" center and cause weight loss.

Therefore you can appreciate how your appetite and weight is controlled by a delicate balance between those factors and the two appetite centers in the brain.

50. WHAT IS A PHYSICIAN SUPERVISED MEDICAL WEIGHT LOSS PROGRAM?

As we discussed previously, obesity is a multifactorial problem and a chronic disease that needs to be addressed by a multidisciplinary team, meaning a team of obesity experts including surgeons and medical specialists.

Medical weight loss is becoming an integral part of any comprehensive weight loss center like we previously discussed. When you are enrolled in a medical weight loss program, the bariatrician (medical obesity expert) will try to find out what are the factors that are contributing to your obesity and assess whether you are ready and motivated to make life style changes in order to lose weight.

Those lifestyle changes usually include diet changes and behavioral changes in addition to enrollment in a structured physical program. The goals of any medical weight loss program will be to improve your health and quality of life in addition to weight loss. Usually bariatricians set an initial goal of 5–10% weight loss.

Many studies have shown that even with 5% weight loss patients feel better and achieve significant improvements in their health and quality of life. An initial goal of 5% is very reasonable and feasible. You may also be seen by a dietitian in order to come up with a meal plan to achieve an energy deficit of 500–800 calories/day; instead of eating an average of 2000 calories per day, the goal would be to eat 1200–1500 calories per day. As for the physical activity, the recommendation is 150–250 minutes per week of moderate intensity. The goal is to start slow and build up over time. Resistance training can be part of a weight loss program and therefore you will be recommended to do 2–3 sessions of resistance training per week.

The most important aspects of any medical weight loss program are consistency and one-on-one counseling. This means frequent sessions and long follow-ups are the norm. We usually recommend at least 14 sessions over 6 months whether one-on-one or in a class format.

All the procedures discussed above are what we call intensive lifestyle intervention. Other forms of intervention can incorporate the use of commercial programs that include meal plans.

The usual weight loss pattern after any program is progressive weight loss for 6 months followed by a plateau and then weight gain. To avoid weight gain the patient is usually counseled on the interventions available to maintain long term weight loss, these include self-monitoring (food recording and self-weighing) in addition to participation in programs that last more than 6 months.

Obviously if your BMI is greater than 35 and you start gaining weight again after the first 6 months you may be referred to see a bariatric surgeon.

CONCLUSION

In conclusion, I hope that you enjoyed this book and found it useful. Before we finish, I would like to emphasize that bariatric surgery is very safe and effective and also has a high success rate. If you suffer from morbid obesity or obesity-related medical conditions you owe it to yourself and your family to consider bariatric surgery.

Bariatric surgery will have a huge positive impact on your life and the life of your family. The main thing to remember is that if you decide to have surgery you need to do some research ahead of time and choose the right surgeon and program in order to have a successful outcome. You also need to remember that surgery is not the easy way out and that you will have to be committed to long-lasting lifestyle changes. You will have to put effort into the process to make sure that you not only lose the weight but also keep the weight off.

Saying that, I would like to wish you good luck and an enjoyable journey toward a healthier and happier you!

Printed in Great Britain
by Amazon